Occupational Therapy Groups for Addressing Mental Health Challenges in School-Aged Populations

A Tier 2 Resource

Occupational Therapy Groups for Addressing Mental Health Challenges in School-Aged Populations

A Tier 2 Resource

Editors

Brad E. Egan, OTD, PhD, CADC, OTR/L

Associate Professor of Occupational Therapy
DePaul University
Chicago, Illinois

Cindy Sears, OTD, MA, OTR/L, BCP

Assistant Professor and Director of Curriculum
Hawai'i Pacific University
Honolulu, Hawai'i

Allen Keener, OTD, MS, OTR/L, ATP

Associate Professor and Doctoral Capstone Coordinator
Eastern Kentucky University
Richmond, Kentucky

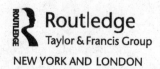

Routledge
Taylor & Francis Group

NEW YORK AND LONDON

pational Therapy Groups for Addressing Mental Health Challenges in School-Aged Populations: A Tier 2 Resource
.des an Instructor's Manual specifically available for faculty use.
e visit http://www.routledge.com/9781630915568 to obtain access.

ublished in 2023 by SLACK Incorporated

hed 2024 by Routledge
nird Avenue, New York, NY 10058

Routledge
Square, Milton Park, Abingdon, Oxon OX14 4RN

·dge is an imprint of the Taylor & Francis Group, an informa business

3 Taylor & Francis Group

y of Congress Cataloging-in-Publication Data

s: Egan, Brad E., editor. | Sears, Cindy, editor. | Keener, Allen, editor.
Occupational therapy groups for addressing mental health challenges in school-aged
ulations : a tier 2 resource / editors, Brad E. Egan, Cindy Sears, Allen Keener.
iption: Thorofare, NJ : SLACK Incorporated, [2023] | Includes
iographical references and index.
fiers: LCCN 2023002004 (print) | ISBN 9781630915568 (paperback) |
cts: MESH: Mental Disorders--rehabilitation | Child Behavior |
·lescent Behavior | Occupational Therapy--methods | School Mental
lth Services | Early Medical Intervention | Case Reports
fication: LCC RJ102 (print) | NLM WS 350.6 |
C 362.2/0425083--dc23/eng/20230315
cord available at https://lccn.loc.gov/2023002004

· Artist: Tinhouse Design

: 9781630915568 (pbk)
: 9781003525318 (ebk)

10.4324/9781003525318

 Additional resources can be found at
http://www.routledge.com/9781630915568

Dedication

This book is especially dedicated to

Reagan and Jason

and

all the occupational therapy practitioners who remain excited and show up ready to respond to the wo
ever-demanding call for action to support participation in meaningful occupation and all the struggi
students who are shouldering the burdens of unmet mental health needs and hold space for hope th
tomorrow may be better than today.

Contents

Contents

Contents

upational Therapy Groups for Addressing Mental Health Challenges in School-Aged Populations: A Tier 2 Resource
udes an Instructor's Manual specifically available for faculty use.
se visit http://www.routledge.com/9781630915568 to obtain access.

About the Editors

Brad E. Egan, OTD, PhD, CADC, OTR/L, is a tenured associate professor of occupational therapy at University and former founding site coordinator and associate professor of occupational therapy at Rhyne University's Columbia, South Carolina campus. He has worked extensively in community-based health with adults and children. He currently enjoys using chess in after-school programming to p mental well-being for at-risk youth. Dr. Egan has been an occupational therapist for 20 years and a ce alcohol and drug counselor for 7 years. His research interests include homelessness, substance use, after programming, the impact of occupation-based interventions on building resilience, and protective facto Egan received his bachelor's degree in Spanish from the University of South Carolina, master's degree in studies from the University of Alabama, a doctoral degree in occupational therapy from Creighton Uni and a PhD in education from Northcentral University. He enjoys coffee around the clock, faux taxiderm casts, and skylines.

Cindy Sears, OTD, MA, OTR/L, BCP, is an assistant professor and director of curriculum at Hawai'i University's Doctor of Occupational Therapy Program in Honolulu, Hawai'i. Prior to this role, she was ar tant professor at Lenoir-Rhyne University's Columbia, South Carolina campus. Cindy has more than 30 y clinical practice in pediatric occupational therapy with 20 years devoted to school systems therapy. She re her American Occupational Therapy Association board certification in pediatrics in 1999 and again in 20 received her undergraduate and doctoral degrees in occupational therapy from the Medical University of Carolina and a master's degree in business from Webster University. Dr. Sears is passionate about occup therapy, mental health, person-centered measurement, and the science of hope. She loves yoga, running, t Walt Disney World, and time spent with her family, her husband, Jeff, and her twin Maltipoos, Tyler and S

Allen Keener, OTD, MS, OTR/L, ATP, was a fifth-grade classroom teacher before becoming an occupa therapist. He has practiced occupational therapy in a variety of settings, including outpatient adults and p rics, skilled nursing, inpatient rehabilitation, acute care, inpatient mental health, home health, and rehab agement. He became certified as an assistive technology professional through the Rehabilitation Engin and Assistive Technology Society of North America in 2017 and maintains assistive technology as a scho interest. Dr. Keener also holds specialty certifications in online course development and teaching and pl agent modalities. Before joining the faculty at Eastern Kentucky University, Dr. Keener was tenured f and director of the occupational therapy assistant program at Wallace State Community College. In 20 received the Alabama Community College System Chancellor's Award of Excellence for his work in the oc tional therapy assistant program at Wallace State and service to the college. In 2019, he was awarded a Na Institute for Staff and Organizational Development Award of Excellence for Teaching and Leadership annual National Institute for Staff and Organizational Development conference in Austin, Texas. His in in occupational therapy include but are not limited to occupation-based practice, teaching and learnin enabling occupation through assistive technology across the lifespan.

Contributing Authors

Molly Bathje, PhD, MS, OTR/L (Sections 1 and 3)
Assistant Professor
College of Science and Health
DePaul University
Chicago, Illinois

Patricia Bowyer, EdD, MS, OTR, FAOTA, SFHEA
(Sections 1 and 3)
Professor and PhD Program Coordinator
School of Occupational Therapy
College Health Sciences
Texas Woman's University
Denton, Texas
Associate Director of Research
Lonestar LEND
Texas Medical Center
Houston, Texas

Stephanie Brauch, MSOT, OTR/L (Section 3)
CaroMont Health Rehab & Sports Medicine
Gastonia, North Carolina

Anna Brown, MS, OTR/L (Sections 1 and 3)
Occupational Therapist
Regional School District 5

Mark Bumgarner, MS (Sections 1 and 3)
Executive Director
Catawba County United Way
Hickory, North Carolina

Susan Cahill, PhD, OTR/L, FAOTA (Section 3)
Director
Evidence-Based Practice
American Occupational Therapy Association
North Bethesda, Maryland

Bobbi Carrlson, PhD, OTR/L (Sections 1 and 3)
Instructor
Department of Occupational Therapy
School of Medicine and Health Sciences
University of North Dakota
Grand Forks, North Dakota

Theresa Carlson Carroll, OTD, OTR/L (Section
Clinical Associate Professor
Valparaiso University
Valparaiso, Indiana

Ray Cendejas, COTA/L (Sections 1 and 3)
Occupational Therapy Assistant
Occupational Therapy Program
Ascension Alexian Brothers Housing and
Health Alliance
Chicago, Illinois

Paula Cook, OTD, OTR/L (Sections 1 and 3)
Occupational Therapist
Summerlin Hospital
Part-Time Instructor
Touro University Nevada
University of Las Vegas
Las Vegas, Nevada

Marcela De La Pava, MS, OTR/L (Sections 1 and
Occupational Therapist
Marcela De La Pava Occupational Therapy, PC
White Plains, New York

Anna Domina, OTD, OTR/L (Sections 1 and 3)
Associate Professor of Occupational Therapy
Department of Occupational Therapy
Creighton University
Omaha, Nebraska

Jerry Dye, Jr., MA, MEd, NCC, LCMHCA-NC
(Section 1)
Mental Health Counselor
Egan Counseling and Consulting
Charlotte, North Carolina

Megan Eads, BSHS, OTD, OTR/L (Section 3)
Assistant Professor
Occupational Therapy Department
Lewis University
Romeoville, Illinois

Esposito, OTD, OTR/L (Section 3)
nd Assistant Professor
nent of Occupational Therapy
ne College
e, New York

Fecht, OTD, OTR/L, BCP (Sections 1 and 3)
r of Academic Clinical Education
sistant Professor
ment of Occupational Therapy
of Pharmacy and Health Professions
on University
, Nebraska

riguglietti, DHA, MA, OTR/L
is 1 and 3)
nic Fieldwork Coordinator
ttional Therapy Program
thtown College
thtown, Pennsylvania

Harris, COTA/L (Sections 1 and 3)
Association for Special Education
age County (SASED)
llinois

.. Heffron, PhD, OTR/L (Sections 1 and 3)
ate Chair and Associate Professor
ment of Occupational Therapy
of Health Sciences and Human Performance
College
New York

Helgesen, OTR/L (Sections 1 and 3)
ork City Department of Education
ork City, New York

Hettlinger, MSOT, OTR/L (Section 3)
ational Therapist
ient Pediatrics
Kids Pediatric Therapy
urles, Illinois

Wilson James, PhD, MPA, PMP, OTR/L, FAOTA
n 3)
ate Professor
l of Occupational Therapy
-Rhyne University
bia, South Carolina

Janet S. Jedlicka, PhD, OTR/L, FAOTA
(Sections 1 and 3)
Professor and Chair
Department of Occupational Therapy
School of Medicine and Health Sciences
University of North Dakota
Grand Forks, North Dakota

Anne Kiraly-Alvarez, OTD, OTR/L, SCSS (Section 3)
Associate Professor and
Director of Capstone Development
Occupational Therapy Program
Midwestern University
Downers Grove, Illinois

Christine Kivlen, PhD, OTR/L (Sections 1 and 3)
Assistant Professor
Health Care Sciences
(Occupational Therapy Program)
Wayne State University
Detroit, Michigan

Toymika LeFlore, MEd, OTR/L (Sections 1 and 3)
Occupational Therapist
Chicago Public Schools
Oak Park, Illinois

Kathryn M. Loukas, OTD, MS, OTR/L, FAOTA
(Sections 1 and 3)
Clinical Professor of Occupational Therapy
Maine LEND Training Director
University of New England
Portland, Maine

Wanda Mahoney, PhD, OTR/L, FAOTA (Section 3)
Associate Professor of Occupational Therapy
and Medicine
Program in Occupational Therapy
School of Medicine
Washington University
St. Louis, Missouri

Anthony (Tony) Mesiano, Jr., MSW, LCSW, BCD,
NCAC-1 (Section 3)
Director of Outpatient Services
Chicago Behavioral Hospital Outpatient Services
Des Plaines, Illinois

Sarah Nielsen, PhD, OTR/L, FAOTA (Sections 1 and 3)
Associate Professor
Occupational Therapy Department
School of Medicine and Health Sciences
University of North Dakota
Grand Forks, North Dakota

Jane Clifford O'Brien, PhD, OTR/L, FAOTA (Section 3)
Professor
Occupational Therapy Department
University of New England
Biddeford, Maine

Jorge Ochoa, OTR/L (Sections 1 and 3)
Founder and Owner
TamboRhythms
San Antonio, Texas

Laurette Olson, PhD, OTR/L, FAOTA
(Sections 1 and 3)
Professor and Program Director
Graduate Occupational Therapy Program
New York-Presbyterian Iona
School of Health Sciences
Iona University
New Rochelle, New York

Linda M. Olson, PhD, OTR/L, FAOTA (Section 1)
Assistant Professor
Department of Occupational Therapy
Rush University
Chicago, Illinois

Gina Rainelli, OTD, OTR/L (Sections 1 and 3)
Occupational Therapist
Capernaum Pediatric Therapy
Richfield, Minnesota

Nashauna (Neki) Richardson, EdD, MS, OTR/L
(Section 3)
Site Coordinator and Assistant Professor
Occupational Therapy Program
Lenoir Rhyne University
Columbia, South Carolina

Teri K. Rupp, MOT, OTR/L, C/NDT (Sections 1
PhD Candidate
Texas Woman's University
Denton, Texas
Auburn School District
Auburn, Washington

Erin Schwier, EdD, OTD, OTR/L (Section 3)
Program Director/Associate Professor
Occupational Therapy Department
University of St. Augustine for Health Sciences
San Marcos, California

Aubrey Sejuit, PhD, LISW-CP, LCAS, MEd, GC
(Section 1)
Assistant Professor of Social Work and Counsel
College of Education and Health Professions
Limestone University
Gaffney, South Carolina

Meaghan Smeraglia, MOT, OTR/L, CCA (Sectio
Occupational Therapist
Inpatient Adolescent Mental Health
UI Health
Chicago, Illinois

Pam Stephenson, OTD, OTR/L, BCP, FAOTA
(Section 3)
Associate Professor
Occupational Therapy Program
Murphy Deming College of Health Sciences
Mary Baldwin University
Staunton, Virginia

Ashley Stoffel, OTD, OTR/L, FAOTA (Section 3)
Clinical Associate Professor
Department of Occupational Therapy
University of Illinois Chicago
Chicago, Illinois

Karen Stornello, OTD, OTR/L (Sections 1 and 3)
Occupational Therapist
School Association for Special Education
in DuPage County
Lisle, Illinois

Suman, OTD, OTR/L, BCP, SCSS (Section 3)
tional Therapist
ille Community Unit School District #203
ille, Illinois

Thinnes, OTD, OTR/L, FNAP
s 1 and 3)
te Professor of Occupational Therapy
ment of Occupational Therapy
on University
, Nebraska

homure, OTD, OTR/L, LCSW
s 1 and 3)
l Assistant Professor
ment of Occupational Therapy
sity of Illinois Chicago
o, Illinois

(Patee) Tomsic, OTD, MS, OTR/L (Section 3)
nt Professor
of Occupational Therapy Program
te University
e, North Carolina

Ingris Treminio, DrOT, OT/L, BCP (Section 3)
Clinical Assistant Professor
Occupational Therapy Department
Florida International University—
Modesto A. Maidique Campus
Miami, Florida

Jeaneen M. Tucker, BS, MEd, EdS (Foreword)
Education Department
University of South Carolina/
Teacher Induction Program
Columbia, South Carolina

Jessica Weiler, OTD, OTR/L, CTRP (Section 3)
Owner
Thrive Therapy LLC
Madison, Wisconsin

Foreword

Public schools are a microcosm of society. The trauma occurring across the United States plays out schools every single day. There is no greater need in our current educational environment than direct s for mental health issues. This need has been evident for years as we have become increasingly desensit the all-too-frequent school shootings and mass murders within our communities. In addition, the COV crisis has dramatically changed the delivery of education and continues to have a palpable negative imp our children, families, and education teams.

I have been an educator for 40 years and served as a special education teacher, guidance counsel school administrator. My career began as a teacher for students labeled "emotionally disturbed." Duri tenure in public education, I have seen this disability expand dramatically, with many students rem unidentified and in dire need of support. This pressing need always guided me to question how we could meet our students' needs.

Dr. Cindy Sears served as an occupational therapist at Round Top Elementary where I was the princi 18.5 years. Our collaboration transformed my education lens! Dr. Sears introduced our already highly suc faculty to the developmental neurologic, sensory, motor, and perceptual foundations for learning, and ho focused approach could directly impact student success. Together, we saw the endless potential of the kno of occupational therapy services for all our students. Through multiple interdisciplinary initiatives, we many supports for students and teachers, including a foundational skills–based morning video series, as a critical thinking lab in which students in Tiers 1, 2, and 3 could benefit by working through educa skill-building stations with the goal of increasing self-awareness, social-emotional regulation, classroo ticipation, performance, and cognitive potential. Our lab gained visitors from across the southeast who to emulate our model as we provided data from successful student case studies.

This text is precisely what is needed for schools today. Sadly, it is rare for any school to have an occupa therapist on site daily; however, the group strategies presented within, when modeled by the school occupa therapist, can be supported by all educators at some level while the occupational therapist is off campus. F the knowledge that the occupational therapist is working directly with the students' needs in the social-em al domain will positively impact the mental health stressors of the classroom teachers, who too often feel h in the face of 25 or more students and unrealistic pacing guides and achievement expectations.

Public schools have long been considered the foundation of our democracy, which we all must admit experiencing an intense destabilization. This text and its rich resources are a must-have for every school United States!

—Jeaneen M. Tucker, BS, ME
South Carolina Council for Exceptional Children Principal of the Year
School Carolina Association of School Administrators Lifetime Achievement Award

Introduction

School settings are the most common place children and youth receive mental health services. Schoo[l] mental health and behavioral health services cost nearly $4 billion dollars annually and represent close of all treatment (Osagiede et al., 2018). Although schools have become the de facto mental health center f[or] dren and youth, many do not have enough trained personnel to adequately meet students' mental healt[h] (Cahill & Egan, 2017a). Strategic service delivery models are necessary to optimize resource use and ma[ximize] the number of students who can be served. Most schools organize mental health services around the health model, which is based on three increasingly intense tiers. Additionally, school-based mental hea[lth ser]vices follow a systematic problem-solving approach that is overseen by a problem-solving team open to di[verse] school professionals, including occupational therapy practitioners (Cahill & Lopez-Reyna, 2013).

The traditional three-tiered model for school-based mental health services is consistent with large school-based program frameworks (e.g., Positive Behavioral Interventions and Supports, Respo[nse to] Intervention [RtI]). Tier 1, also referred to as the universal level, offers mental health supports to all st[udents.] These school-wide interventions focus on mental health promotion, social-emotional learning, and su[pport]ing positive social interactions. Universal screening is typically completed in Tier 1, and 80% of stude[nts are] expected to have screening results that indicate they are thriving and expected to benefit solely from this [tier of] services (Cahill & Egan, 2017b). The remaining 20% of students are expected to need targeted Tier 2 and [inten]sive Tier 3 supportive services to address screening results indicative of mental health concerns. Tier 2 st[udents] (15%) present with issues and screening results that categorize them as languishing and being at-risk for [mental] health challenges. Students in need of Tier 2 supports are typically good candidates for early interven[ing ser]vices usually provided in a small group format. Tier 2 group interventions are focused on providing just-i[n-time] targeted support to address internalizing and externalizing behaviors and to prevent or delay the studen[t from] meeting the diagnostic criteria for a mental health disorder. Those students who meet the criteria for a [mental] illness or who have already been diagnosed with a mental disorder represent the 5% who may benefi[t from] intensive services. Services at this level are justifiably individualized and closely monitor changes (both p[ositive] and negative) in symptoms and reports of subjective well-being (Cahill & Egan, 2017b).

Occupational therapy practitioners have a rich history of working in traditional mental health se[ttings.] Their contributions and role in serving school-based mental health needs has grown over the past [decade] and continues to grow. According to an American Occupational Therapy Association position stateme[nt on] mental health recovery (2016), school systems practice was identified as a key mental health practice s[etting.] Occupational therapy practitioners are uniquely positioned in schools to support the development, pro[vision,] and monitoring of interventions designed to meet the mental and behavioral health needs of students en[rolled] in special education and general education. In a study by Cahill and Egan (2017a), a small group of [school] psychologists and social workers (traditional mental health providers) completed several online module[s and] discussions about how occupational therapy professionals could support students' mental health promotio[n and] prevention needs. **They unanimously concluded that occupational therapists should be doing more an[d saw] great value in occupation-based group interventions for students receiving Tier 2 and Tier 3 school-[based] mental health services.**

Calls to action within the profession and legislative changes have created opportunities and cont[inued] momentum among occupational therapy practitioners to not only assess but *actually address* the mental [health] needs of school-aged children with occupation-based interventions. For example, while serving as Am[erican] Occupational Therapy Association vice president, Dr. Ginny Stoffel strategically increased the profession's [focus] on mental health and called on practitioners to consider addressing the countless opportunities in scho[ol sys]tems practice to apply our specialized knowledge and skills in mental health and to possibly regain our fo[oting] as qualified mental health providers. Dr. Susan Cahill repeatedly encouraged occupational therapy practiti[oners] to join school-based problem-solving teams to support behavioral and mental health needs of general e[duca]tion students (e.g., Cahill, 2010; Cahill et al., 2008; Cahill & Lopez-Reyna, 2013) and developed the Fra[me of] Reference for School-Aged Children with Anxiety and Depression (Cahill, 2020) to support school-based [inter]ventions for kids with symptoms of anxiety and depression. Legislatively, there has been strong federal su[pport] for school-based mental health programs and services. Occupational therapy practitioners were named e[ligible]

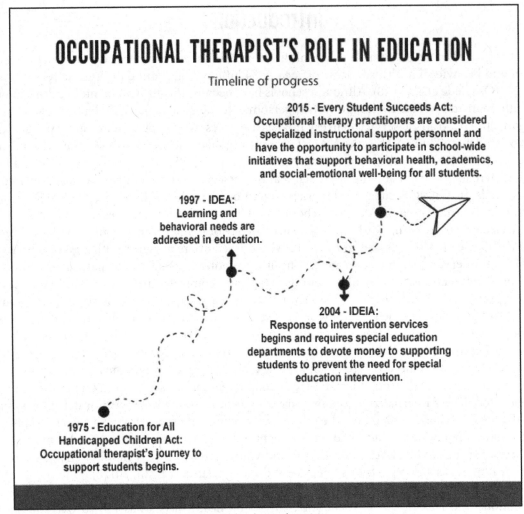

Figure I-1. Timeline of occupational therapist's role in education.

specialized instructional support personnel in the Every Student Succeeds Act for their specialized skills ining in providing tiered interventions. Among the prioritized tasks mentioned for specialized instruc-support personnel was providing school-based mental health services and interventions that addressed -wide mental illness prevention, resiliency-building, individual and group counseling, and collaboration ommunity-based mental health providers and services (National Alliance of Specialized Instructional rt Personnel, 2019).

e calls to action are being answered (Figure I-1). Occupational therapy practitioners in school systems practice emained focused on addressing the mental health needs of students in special education and have recently orking hard to fill a critical service gap in addressing the mental health needs of students in general educa-s such, there is much to celebrate professionally at the Tier 1 level. A systematic review of occupational therapy ntions focused on mental health prevention and promotion for children and youth found strong effects for ting school-wide social-emotional learning, bullying prevention, and stress management (Arbesman et al., Dr. Susan Bazyk's tireless work in supporting mental health promotion has forged a very strong community tice within school systems practice and an equally strong occupational therapist–led program, Every Moment s. Specifically, a 6-week Comfortable Cafeteria intervention, which is part of Every Moment Counts, indicated cally significant improvements for students across critical mental health and positive school climate factors

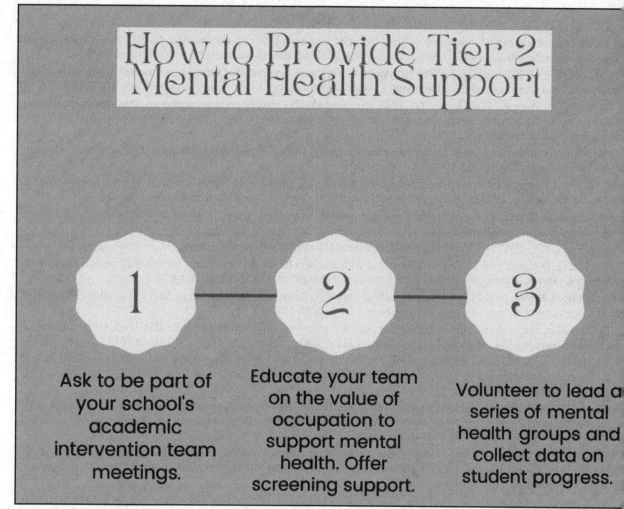

How to Provide Tier 2 Mental Health Support

1 Ask to be part of your school's academic intervention team meetings.

2 Educate your team on the value of occupation to support mental health. Offer screening support.

3 Volunteer to lead a series of mental health groups and collect data on student progress.

Figure I-2. How to provide Tier 2 occupational therapy services to support mental health.

(Bazyk et al., 2018). Another successful and popular Tier 1 program developed by an occupational therapist Kuypers, is the Zones of Regulation. The Zones of Regulation program focuses on skills to support emotion self-regulation. It has been adopted widely by clinicians from different professional backgrounds and has been i mented successfully in large groups and classroom-wide general education settings (McQuaid, 2018).

Despite more concerted school mental health programs and services, mental health concerns con to increase at alarming rates among adolescents and youth, particularly with respect to mood disorder suicide-related issues (Twenge et al., 2019). These data, along with anticipated worries about the effects pandemic on school-aged children and youth, invite a stronger call to intervene as early as possible to de eliminate a mental health disorder through targeted and trauma-responsive Tier 2 interventions. Unfortur a review of school-based mental health programs suggested that schools tend to lack systematic process identifying students for Tier 2 programs, sufficient resources and time to plan Tier 2 interventions, and ade support (Moore et al., 2019). This same study found that schools without robust Tier 2 supports often ha other choice than to put additional pressure on special education services and related providers (Moore 2019). For this reason, we have chosen to focus this text exclusively on Tier 2 issues and interventions, ar hope that this toolbox will serve you well as you grow your Tier 2 practice and further strengthen your and Tier 3 interventions (Figure I-2).

ences

n Occupational Therapy Association. (2016). *Occupational therapy's role with mental health recovery*. www.aota. media/Corporate/Files/AboutOT/Professionals/WhatIsOT/MH/Facts/Mental%20Health%20Recovery.pdf.

n, M., Bazyk, S., & Nochajski, S. M. (2013). Systematic review of occupational therapy and mental health promotion, ntion, and intervention for children and youth. *American Journal of Occupational Therapy, 67*(6), e120-e130.

., Demirjian, L., Horvath, F., & Doxsey, L. (2018). The comfortable cafeteria program for promoting student participa-nd enjoyment: An outcome study. *American Journal of Occupational Therapy, 72*(3), 7203205050p1-7203205050p9. //doi.org/10.5014/ajot.2018.025379

. M. (2010). Contributions made by occupational therapists in RtI: A pilot study. *Journal of Occupational Therapy,* ls, & Early Intervention, 3*(1), 3-10.

. M. (2020). A frame of reference for school-aged children with anxiety and depression. In P. Kramer, J. Hinojoa, & T. e (Eds.), *Frames of reference for pediatric occupational therapy* (pp. 523-554). Wolters Kluwer.

. M., & Egan, B. E. (2017a). Perceptions of occupational therapy involvement in school mental health: A pilot study. *Journal of Occupational Therapy, 5*(1), 5.

. M., & Egan, B. E. (2017b). Identifying youth with mental health conditions at school. *OT Practice, 22*(5), 1-7.

. M., Holt, C., & Cassidy, M. (2008). Collaborating with teachers to support student achievement through early inter-ng services. *Journal of Occupational Therapy, Schools, & Early Intervention, 1*(3-4), 263-270.

. M., & Lopez-Reyna, N. (2013). Expanding school-based problem-solving teams to include occupational therapists. al of Occupational Therapy, Schools, & Early Intervention, 6*(4), 314-325.

d, E. (2018). Feasibility study: Implementing the zones of regulation® curriculum at a whole-class level. *American Journal cupational Therapy, 72*(4 Suppl. 1), 7211505083p1-7211505083p1. https://doi.org/10.5014/ajot.2018.72S1-PO1014

S. A., Mayworm, A. M., Stein, R., Sharkey, J. D., & Dowdy, E. (2019). Languishing students: Linking complete mental h screening tools in schools to Tier 2 intervention. *Journal of Applied School Psychology, 35*(3), 257-289. https://doi. 0.1080/15377903.2019.1577780

l Alliance of Specialized Instruction Support Personnel. (2019). *National Alliance of Specialized Instructional Support nnel effective specialized instructional support services* (Research Brief). Retrieved from www.nasisp.org/wp-content/ ads/2021/03/NASISPResearchDoc2019.pdf

le, O., Costa, S., Spaulding, A., Rose, J., Allen, K. E., Rose, M., & Apatu, E. (2018). Teachers' perceptions of student men-ealth: The role of school-based mental health services delivery model. *Children & Schools, 40*(4), 240-248. https://doi. 0.1093/cs/cdy020

, J. M., Cooper, A. B., Joiner, T. E., Duffy, M. E., & Binau, S. G. (2019). Age, period, and cohort trends in mood disorder ators and suicide-related outcomes in a nationally representative dataset, 2005-2017. *Journal of Abnormal Psychology,* 3), 185-199. https://doi.org/10.1037/abn0000410

How to Use This Book

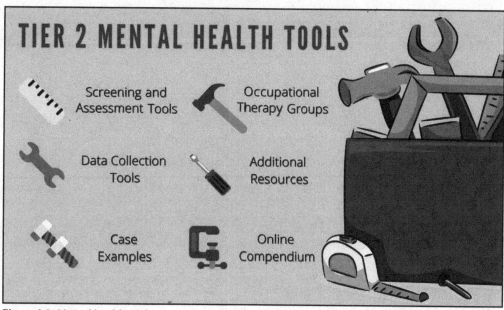

Figure I-3. Mental health tools.

Occupational Therapy Groups for Addressing Mental Health Challenges in School-Aged Populations: A Resource was designed with occupational therapy practitioners in mind to support their efforts in expandi role of occupational therapy practitioners in school systems practice (Figure I-3). The activities in this to are written with a Tier 2 intention and can be easily scaled down for Tier 1 initiatives and scaled up for interventions. We have put together a variety of creative ideas and tools that can support practitioners in j their school's problem-solving team (if they have not done so already) and their efforts to fully meet the r health needs of students. Although this toolbox was designed for occupational therapy practitioners in s systems practice, this text can be of great use for students in occupational therapy/occupational therapy ass programs, educators in occupational therapy/occupational therapy assistant programs, and our colleag other professions who work every day to meet the mental health needs of students.

This book is divided into five sections, each offering a unique Tier 2 tool. The five sections are:

1. Case Examples

   These cases provide an opportunity to review internalizing and externalizing behaviors, consider stre and examine issues impacting occupational performance.

2. Screening and Assessment Tools

   This section provides a quick overview of free or low-cost screening tools and assessments that may be to inform Tier 2 decisions.

3. Occupational Therapy Groups

   This section offers a variety of occupation-based and occupation-focused small group interventions. group comes with suggested processing questions and a related summary note form.

4. Data Collection Tools

   This section contains example data tracking templates that may help to monitor the outcomes of interventions.

5. Additional Resources

   This section includes various links to references, resources, and miscellaneous forms that can help to your school mental health practice.

t, we invite all readers to use their own creativity to customize these tools for their own practice! Feel adapt any of these tools to meet your client's age, occupational needs, developmental capacity, and/or mental constraints.

Sincerely,
Brad, Cindy, and Allen

Section 1

Case Examples

Egan, B. E., Sears, C., & Keener, A. (Eds.). *Occupational Therapy Groups for*
Mental Health Challenges in School-Aged Populations: A Tier 2 Resource
© 2023 Taylor & Fran

Introduction to the Cases

Most often, potential mental health issues present in school and classroom settings as internalizing and nalizing behaviors. Externalizing behaviors tend to be outwardly visible and disruptive. As such, they usual the attention of teachers and staff. Internalizing behaviors, in contrast, are directed inwardly and are often in to others. Unfortunately, it is far too common for a student with internalizing behaviors to stay under the and never receive services or receive them only after they have become extremely distressed. To serve st Tier 2 needs, it is important to be able to identify externalizing and internalizing behaviors and understan they impact occupational performance and participation at school. These cases are meant to provide oppo ties for you to review these behaviors, while also considering personal strengths and occupational informa

The American Occupational Therapy Association's school mental health work group has advocated f illustrated the benefits of a strength-based approach to supporting learners in both general education and education. A strengths-based orientation aids the occupational therapy practitioner in designing interve that provide opportunities to better understand and use one's personal strengths. Identifying personal str is critical to promoting hope, increasing self-efficacy, and supporting recovery. To encourage continued p with identifying strengths, the editors intentionally provided a blank three-bulleted list for each case. It is th that users of the resource will be able to identify even more than three strengths in each vignette.

Tier 2 Elementary School Case #1: *Annie*

Sarah Nielsen, PhD, OTR/L, FAOTA; Janet S. Jedlicka, PhD, OTR/L, FAOTA;
and Bobbi Carrlson, PhD, OTR/L

DENT STRENGTHS

ifying personal strengths is critical to promoting hope, increasing self-efficacy, and supporting recovery. To encourage
nued practice with identifying strengths, the editors intentionally provided a blank three-bulleted list for each case. It is
ope that users of the resource will be able to identify even more than three strengths in each vignette.)

CUPATIONAL NEEDS

HOOL BARRIERS: INTERNALIZING BEHAVIORS

Social isolation

Unsuccessful cooperative group work

Limited peer interactions

Declining academic performance

RSONAL FACTOR CONSIDERATIONS

Single-parent home

Parents' impending divorce

Limited financial resources

Bullying from peers

Shy

Only one identified friend

Client Report

Annie is a 10-year-old girl who is a fourth grader at Roosevelt Elementary School, where she start
kindergartener. Annie's typical routine begins with her mother dropping her off for before-school progra
at 7:15 AM. She is in one classroom with 22 students and attends physical education and music class out
her homeroom. She attends after-school programming until 6:00 PM, when her mother picks her up. Her
has recently raised concerns with the academic intervention team about Annie not engaging with her peer
given cooperative tasks. Her grades have subsequently slipped, and her mom is also concerned.

Annie reported that she likes school, but she does not like working with other students on projects.
ported that she usually gets good grades on assignments. She knows she has not been doing as well with
assignments lately, which upsets her. Her grades in science and social studies have declined the most, esp
on partner assignments. Annie wishes she could just do assignments on her own. Her teacher reported s
observed Annie sitting with her arms crossed if her ideas are not used. Annie stated that her peers never l
ideas and that they say they are "stupid." On one occasion, Annie refused to do the group assignment and te
teacher she wanted to do it alone, but her teacher said no. Annie reported she has one friend, but she does
tend her school. Annie's teacher also reported that Annie tends to play alone on the playground.

Annie lives at home with her mom and one older brother, 6 years her senior. Last Christmas, Ann
brother, and her mom returned home from church service to find that Annie's dad had moved out and take
his belongings. He moved in with another woman and her children, both of whom are in elementary schoc
their recent affair. He has not paid any child support or visited Annie since Christmas. Annie's mom now
double shifts as a nurse assistant to support the family.

Annie's mom reported that Annie has met all her developmental milestones and has done well in sch
this point. She is independent in self-care, only needing reminders occasionally to complete these tasks. At
she watches television and plays on her tablet. She is shy and only has one friend outside of school. She
rigid at times about how things are done, and this can cause difficulties within her family life and when the
has to make decisions together. For example, if the family is going out to eat and selecting a location, Ann
often shut down and refuse to eat if her choice is not selected. Annie's mom feels she should have outgrow
response by now. Annie reported that her mom tells her school is important and she needs to improve her g

Annie also reports enjoying reading and especially likes Beverly Cleary's *Ramona* series. She likes go
the public library. She attended weekly story time at the library once but quit because she said she did not li
children in the group. Her mom has encouraged her to try other organized activities, but Annie has refuse
has requested a cellphone, but her mom has indicated that she cannot have a cellphone because they cannot
one and she is too young. She is not active on social media platforms and reports some of her classmates a
that they think she is "weird" because she does not have a phone or social media accounts.

Tier 2 Elementary School Case #2: _Robert_

Jorge Ochoa, OTR/L

STUDENT STRENGTHS

Identifying personal strengths is critical to promoting hope, increasing self-efficacy, and supporting recovery. To encourage continued practice with identifying strengths, the editors intentionally provided a blank three-bulleted list for each case. It is our hope that users of the resource will be able to identify even more than three strengths in each vignette.)

OCCUPATIONAL NEEDS

SCHOOL BARRIERS: INTERNALIZING BEHAVIORS

Limited work completion

Late assignments and tardiness for class and crossing guard responsibilities

Self-imposed social isolation

Low self-esteem

Declining academic performance

PERSONAL FACTOR CONSIDERATIONS

Affluent family

Parents' high expectations

High-achieving siblings

Somatic symptoms owing to anxiety and stress

Perfectionism paralysis

Increased anxiety and fear of failing

Fear of transitioning to middle school

Client Report

Robert, age 10 years, is a fifth grader at J.K. Williams Elementary school. He has attended Williams Elem
since kindergarten. He lives at home with both parents and an older sibling. His sister, Deborah, attends
High School and is in the 10th grade. She is an all-star softball player and is being recruited nationally for
scholarships. She plays travel ball and recently their dad is gone most weekends to take her to games and
softball scouting events. Robert's mother is a partner at a successful law firm and his father is a computer en
Both speak highly on the importance of education and good grades. They report they do not expect Ro
always get As but do expect him to try his best.

Robert has previously enjoyed walking to school with his friends, and he is proud of his role as a c
guard that requires both before- and after-school responsibilities. His favorite subject is science, and he fre
answers and asks questions in class. He has become somewhat of a teacher's assistant by offering to distribu
pick up classroom supplies. Overall, Robert is an A or B student in his classes. During recess, he is usual
playing dodgeball with his classmates.

Robert's behavior at school has changed during the past 2 months. He is turning in late assignments
not complete them. He rarely studies for tests and falls asleep at his desk often. Grades are also falling to th
D level. He no longer participates in science and has asked the teacher if she could ask someone else to dis
supplies. He is constantly late for his crossing guard duties. He has also withdrawn from his friends; he cho
sit alone during lunch and recess.

When questioned by one of his teachers as to why his behavior has changed or if something is wro
shrugs his shoulders and says that he is just tired all the time and does not want to talk about it. Owing to he
cern, a referral was made to the school counselor. During the meeting, he admitted to the counselor that
nervous about going to middle school the next year and misses his dad since he is now gone most weeken
believes that, even though he has a history of good grades, he always felt that he was not as smart or as suc
as the other students in his class. Robert constantly compares himself with others and becomes anxious v
difficult assignment arises.

He anticipates increased difficulties in middle school. He is constantly afraid of failure and has lo
esteem. He confessed that he was always "stressed out," but he learned to hide it well. Because it is 2 month
the end of the school year, his worries are intensifying. Robert was also concerned that he was disappointi
parents with his lower grades. He is so tired because his sleep routine has been disrupted since he was w
during the night and early in the morning with an anxious or panicked feeling and upset stomach. Therefo
now has a difficult time concentrating on his school work. Toward the end of the meeting, he told the cou
he wished that he had more self-confidence and less stress so that he could enjoy school. Robert's mother i
driving him to and from school to avoid walking with his friends. She feels guilty working long hours and
sure about how to help Robert.

Tier 2 Elementary School Case #3: *Shiloh*

Kelsey Helgesen, OTR/L

DENT STRENGTHS

tifying personal strengths is critical to promoting hope, increasing self-efficacy, and supporting recovery. To encourage
nued practice with identifying strengths, the editors intentionally provided a blank three-bulleted list for each case. It is
ope that users of the resource will be able to identify even more than three strengths in each vignette.)

CUPATIONAL NEEDS

HOOL BARRIERS: INTERNALIZING BEHAVIORS

Selective mutism

Impulsively wandering around the classroom

Difficulty following directions and completing tasks independently

Scribbling on class assignments

Social isolation

Limited academic participation

Referral to the academic intervention team for consideration for special education testing for autism
spectrum disorder

RSONAL FACTOR CONSIDERATIONS

History of sexual abuse

Mother with intellectual delays

Poverty

Client Report

Shiloh, a 6-year-old girl, is a first-grader at a public elementary school in a high-poverty neighborh New York City. Shiloh just began attending this school in the fall and is in a general education class with 1 students. Shiloh's typical school day routine involves taking the school bus, eating free school breakfast in t eteria once she arrives, participating in academic and related arts classes, and taking the bus home at the the day. When Shiloh started at this school, she would not talk to anyone owing to selective mutism. Shilo speaks to familiar adults in the education setting, although she usually speaks quietly in a whisper.

Recently, Shiloh has started to demonstrate some impulsive behaviors in the classroom, such as takin room supplies off of other students' desks; during lessons, she gets out of her seat frequently. She has also sta demonstrate behaviors such as scribbling on her work and laughing inappropriately with no apparent pre event.

Shiloh is a good reader and is very proud that she has started to learn to read this year. She has made academic progress over the past 2 months of the school year. Shiloh has also developed closer friendshi she is more comfortable talking to a few peers. She is also an amazing artist, a talent she has demonstrate kindergarten. She enjoys drawing her favorite television and movie characters and does so with great skill. S reports enjoying going to the movies and shopping with her mom.

Shiloh lives with her mother and two brothers in an apartment building with social services, becau mother has an intellectual disability. She also has several pets, including a puppy. Shiloh's older brother is ir grade in a more restrictive special education setting owing to extreme behaviors and difficulty with emo regulation. Shiloh's younger brother is in general education kindergarten at a different school. She speaks of her younger brother, her mom, and her grandmother, who does not live with them but often takes Shil her younger brother on outings on the weekend. Shiloh used to talk frequently about her dad but has not s much of him during the last few months. She has not given details about the situation, except to say that s not seen him in a while. Her mother's boyfriend of the past 2 years often babysits Shiloh and her younger b and began sexually abusing her over the last 9 months. No one is currently aware of the abuse. Shiloh sa spends most of her time at home playing with her younger brother, watching television, and playing on her Her mom reports that she is very talkative at home and can be verbally aggressive to her mom, which is a be that Shiloh has never engaged in at school. In art class, there was some concern when Shiloh began to draw drawings and captions. Shiloh's family had Child Protective Services involvement when she was a toddler bu not currently have an open case.

Shiloh is generally well-groomed at school, but occasionally she will come in appearing as though he has not been brushed in a few days. If a classroom adult tells her to ask her mom to do her hair, it usually brushed the next day. Her clothes are always clean; recently, she has new clothes, which she has started to poi to classroom adults and seems to take pride in them.

Tier 2 Elementary School Case #4: _Natalia_

Andrea Thinnes, OTD, OTR/L, FNAP
and Anna Domina, OTD, OTR/L

DENT STRENGTHS

ifying personal strengths is critical to promoting hope, increasing self-efficacy, and supporting recovery. To encourage
nued practice with identifying strengths, the editors intentionally provided a blank three-bulleted list for each case. It is
ope that users of the resource will be able to identify even more than three strengths in each vignette.)

CUPATIONAL NEEDS

HOOL BARRIERS: INTERNALIZING BEHAVIORS

Exhausted in school owing to disrupted sleep routine

Difficulty focusing in the classroom

Late and missing class assignments

Inconsistent academic performance

RSONAL FACTOR CONSIDERATIONS

Grief

Fear of dying

Poor self-image → high body mass index

Death of her mother

Father in prison

Lives with aunt and uncle

Client Report

Natalia is a 9-year-old fourth grader at Saratoga Elementary School. She has an older sister, Bethany, 15 years old and a sophomore in high school. She has an older brother, Nicco, who is 11 years old and i grade. Currently, Natalia and her siblings live with their aunt and uncle. The children's mother died 18 mon from a heart attack. After she passed away, their father chose to work day and night at his company to avoid home, in an effort to forget his wife was no longer there. Three months after she passed away, he was fired fr job and charged with fraud and embezzlement from his business partner. After the court found him guilty, sentenced to 15 years in jail. The children chose to live with their favorite aunt and uncle, who live in thei hometown and have two grown children already out of the house.

Natalia's daily routine includes sleeping in until the last minute possible in the morning and then gr a breakfast pastry and fruit juice on her way out the door to catch the school bus. She receives school-pr lunches but tends to eat her friends' leftovers because she still feels hungry. Natalia enjoys several after- clubs. She participates in debate club, ceramics club, and a creative writing group after school 3 days a we eats an after-school snack on the bus ride home, usually chips or sugary snacks and soda. For dinner, he tries to make family dinner time a priority and each child takes a turn cooking dinner with her once each w the evening, they watch television as a family. Natalia spends lots of time also looking on the adopt-a-pet website for a pet the family could adopt.

Natalia describes herself as an animal lover, creative, and social. She has friends at school that are in th clubs but rarely are they allowed to come to her house because other parents are uncomfortable with thei dren associating with her family outside of school. Family is very important to Natalia, especially her siblin aunt and uncle, who have supported them. Natalia has had an increasingly difficult time this school year w her mom. She has gained more weight and has a hard time choosing clothing she is comfortable wearing. S a poor self-image and has a fear of dying young, as her mother did. She often avoids going to sleep until utterly exhausted owing to bedtime fears and thinking about how much she misses her mom. She is grievi loss of her mom and the loss of her family home, and she has resentment toward her father for lying, stealin abandoning the family.

Natalia had been successful in school before her mother's death. The school counselor and teachers hav involved in her grief counseling. Teachers are reporting increasing concerns with Natalia's academic perfor owing to her exhaustion during class, distractibility, and missing and late assignments.

During the school health screenings for the last 2 years, Natalia has had a body mass index of 96%, a school nurse has recommended to Natalia's aunt that a nutrition and healthy lifestyle plan be put in plac grades have declined during fourth grade. Overall, considering the circumstances, Natalia is a hardworkin student and enjoys her friends and teacher.

Tier 2 Elementary School Case #5: *Amena*

Christine Kivlen, PhD, OTR/L
and Jenna L. Heffron, PhD, OTR/L

DENT STRENGTHS

ifying personal strengths is critical to promoting hope, increasing self-efficacy, and supporting recovery. To encourage
nued practice with identifying strengths, the editors intentionally provided a blank three-bulleted list for each case. It is
ope that users of the resource will be able to identify even more than three strengths in each vignette.)

UPATIONAL NEEDS

HOOL BARRIERS: INTERNALIZING BEHAVIORS

Decreased participation in classroom roles and routines

Social isolation during lunch and recess

Missed instructional time owing to somatic symptoms and health room visits

Tardy and missed instruction in physical education

Poor problem-solving skills

Poor self-advocacy

RSONAL FACTOR CONSIDERATIONS

Increased anxiety

Bullied at school

Extended family live in Syria and connect with Amena via Zoom

Member of a marginalized population in the community → Muslim

Client Report

Amena is a second-grade 7-year-old girl at West Utica Elementary, where she has attended school sin
dergarten. Her family is of the middle socioeconomic class, affording their family the ability to send Am
daycare while both of her parents work full time. Amena's typical daily routine includes her mother assistir
her morning rituals, riding the bus to school, attending school from 8:45 AM to 3:00 PM, and attending c
until 6:00 PM, where she is picked up by her dad. As Amena has progressed from kindergarten through
grade, concerns related to anxiety, problem-solving, and social isolation have become more apparent.

Amena's participation has decreased significantly in the classroom. Her teacher, Mrs. White, asked h
she has not been participating or raising her hand very often in class and she responded with, "They gigg
laugh when I talk in class." Mrs. White explained the children are not laughing at her; however, Amena dc
seem to believe her teacher. Mrs. White is also concerned with Amena isolating herself during lunch and
activities. During lunch, Amena is often found sitting alone. Amena reports, "Sometimes Sarah or Becky a
to sit with them, but I know they do not really want me to and will probably just laugh at me." Mrs. White re
out to Amena's daycare attendant regarding how she interacts with her peers outside of the school enviror
and daycare personnel reported similar behaviors.

Additionally, Mrs. White has voiced concerns about Amena's frequent requests to visit the nurse when t
an unexpected event or transition during the school day. Amena will report feeling sick to her stomach, as
show blushing and hives during these requests. Amena has also been withdrawing from physical education
ties. Her teacher reports she is often tardy and less engaged in the activities, particularly those pertaining tc
games. Amena reports, "My favorite part of the school day is going to specials, but I do not like gym."

Amena excels in art and music specials, and her teacher reports above-average skills in English and lar
courses. Many of the adult figures in Amena's life describe her to be pleasant and organized. Mrs. White r
exceptional skills in keeping her desk and school spaces organized. Amena has stated that she loves to learn,
to do well in school, and desires to have friends. She reports being happiest when she is engaging in activitie
as crafts, drawing, painting, and gardening.

Amena also often talks about how much she loves her family. Her parents report she asks questions
her Muslim religion and practices that her family in Syria engages in. Although Amena does not show e
interest in communicating with her peers, she really enjoys using her computer to Zoom and communicat
her extended family in Syria. She is fascinated with every aspect of her extended family's life from the wa
dress to what they eat and the religious events they participate in. Amena often tells her parents, "I wish they
by where we live. I am different than the kids that go to my school." Her parents are concerned that Amer
continue to withdraw at school and have expressed to her teacher how important it is to build connection
social skills to interact with her peers.

Her parents have shared personal information with her teachers and daycare attendants regarding con
tions that have occurred at home. Her parents shared that, although Amena has difficulty engaging with pee
feels more comfortable interacting in small groups. She told her parents, "I share my ideas with Jenny, Fion
Billy who sit in my group, but it's too hard in front of the whole class." Amena has also expressed to her paren
she enjoys spending recess time by herself and feels much better when she goes back to class. Amena and her
ily are hopeful that she can build upon strong language skills, as well as creative and artistic talents, to foste
sonal self-awareness and self-knowledge, further laying the foundation for self-determination and self-advc

Tier 2 Elementary School Case #6: *Colby*

Anna Brown, MS, OTR/L
and Kathryn M. Loukas, OTD, MS, OTR/L, FAOTA

DENT STRENGTHS

tifying personal strengths is critical to promoting hope, increasing self-efficacy, and supporting recovery. To encourage nued practice with identifying strengths, the editors intentionally provided a blank three-bulleted list for each case. It is ope that users of the resource will be able to identify even more than three strengths in each vignette.)

CUPATIONAL NEEDS

HOOL BARRIERS: EXTERNALIZING BEHAVIORS

Poor academic performance

Poor motor control and motor planning skills; teachers report Colby is "clumsy" and frequently trips and falls

Poor cooperative behavior in the classroom, especially with nonpreferred tasks

Difficulty with activity transitions

Poor participation and cooperative behaviors during physical education and recess

Poor peer relationships

Impulsivity

Overreaction to unexpected situations

Difficulty with behavior regulation, especially self-calming

RSONAL FACTOR CONSIDERATIONS

Trauma

Attention-deficit/hyperactivity disorder (ADHD) and fetal alcohol syndrome

Lives with supportive adoptive parents

Loves blocks, LEGO (The LEGO Group) pieces, and beginner origami

Client Report

   Colby is a 6-year-old boy in the first grade. Colby enjoys being a helper to adults and has strong solita
skills. Colby enjoys toys that he can stack and build with. Colby is motivated to complete activities of daily
tasks, follow directions, and play with peers.

   Colby is below grade level in all academic subjects. Colby has a history of significant outburst behavio
have impacted his ability to access his education. These behaviors include yelling, distractibility, and impu
Colby's behaviors are due to a history of trauma. Colby was removed from his biological parents at the
5 years and was recently adopted. Colby's diagnoses include ADHD and fetal alcohol syndrome. Colby st
with gross motor planning and often seems to be clumsy. Colby has stated his peers make him feel "stup
their comments about his tripping, falling, and bumping into objects. His behavioral outbursts are signif
increased during recess, gym, and times of transition. He yells to avoid a transition or nonpreferred activity
the demands may be set too high or he feels he will be targeted by peers. Colby does seek relationships wit
and struggles to maintain relationships.

   Colby enjoys building with blocks, LEGO pieces, and doing beginner origami. Colby will often choose
these activities when given a choice. He has a difficult time transitioning away from these activities to move
educational or social demands. Colby benefits from visual schedules and timers, close staff proximity, and w
with preferred and trusted adults.

   When engaging with peers, completing classroom work, or playing on the playground, Colby overre
peer and adult interactions. Colby becomes overly loud, moves too quickly, and becomes unable to calm h
These behaviors contribute to an increase in tripping, stumbling, and bumping into objects. Teachers report
enjoys and prefers to be with his peers, but he gets "silly" and "overly excited" when he starts to play with th

   At home, Colby keeps to himself and does not interact often with his younger brother. His parents repo
split toys between different rooms to limit conflicts. Colby's adoptive parents have successfully implemented
of the same visual supports and routines that Colby accesses at school. They also use timers and reminders
activities are about to end. A goal of the family is to have everyone sit at the table together during meals. C
role in the home includes simple chores, such as bringing his plate to the sink and throwing away snack wr
and other trash items. Colby is expected to get himself dressed once his clothes have been laid out and to
his teeth.

Tier 2 Elementary School Case #7: *Dinah*

Paula Cook, OTD, OTR/L
and Ashley Fecht, OTD, OTR/L, BCP

‌DENT STRENGTHS

‌ifying personal strengths is critical to promoting hope, increasing self-efficacy, and supporting recovery. To encourage ‌nued practice with identifying strengths, the editors intentionally provided a blank three-bulleted list for each case. It is ‌ope that users of the resource will be able to identify even more than three strengths in each vignette.)

‌CUPATIONAL NEEDS

‌HOOL BARRIERS: EXTERNALIZING BEHAVIORS

‌Decreased social skill interactions

‌Bullying

‌Suspicious of others

‌Lying and accusatory

‌Fear obsessions limiting attention and focus

‌RSONAL FACTOR CONSIDERATIONS

‌Secondary trauma → brother held at gunpoint

‌Anxiety and fear perseveration

‌High-achieving siblings

Client Report

Dinah is a fifth-grade student at Emilio Escalada Elementary School in Las Vegas, Nevada. She is 1... old and has five siblings: two older brothers (17 and 15 years old), an older sister (12 years old), and two y... sisters (8 and 7 years old). She has lived in Las Vegas her entire life. Her mother is a dental hygienist and her... is a high school biology teacher. A typical day for Dinah includes walking to school with her younger siblin... older siblings attend the local middle and high schools. She plays on the playground for a morning recess... the first bell and then follows her class schedule. Dinah enjoys making friendship bracelets, reading my... writing short stories, and drawing in her notepad. She recently showed an interest in bird watching. She a... joys going to the park district pool to swim. Her parents' work schedules mostly align with her school sc... but there is 1 hour after school every day where Dinah is responsible for watching her younger two siblin... texts her parents when they arrive home.

Six months ago, Dinah's 17-year-old brother was held at gunpoint. The assault happened in the parking... the natural history museum, where her brother works part-time. Her brother was not physically injured but... riences some flashbacks of the event. Dinah has heard her brother retell his escape story many times and... the details about how he ran away from the scene, ran into the museum for help, and was put in a quasi-loc... in the museum office. Her brother said he has seen the assaulter near the museum before, walking to an... a "tent city" where the local homeless population sets up tents. Before this incident, Dinah has visited the... counselor to help with anxiety within the school setting. Her older siblings always excelled in school, and D... grades are average; she struggles with feeling as though she is constantly compared to them.

She has spoken with the school counselor about her brother's experience and expressed that she di... anyone she suspects to be homeless. She began excluding friends of a lower socioeconomic status from her... ground activities. Recently, the teacher noticed this pattern and discussed the issue with the school cou... There is one girl in her class who lives in a hotel; Dinah accused her of stealing her headphones and colore... Later, Dinah learned that her younger siblings had taken her colored pens and she found her headphones... locker. Another time, she confided in her teacher that she was scared that the classmate who lives in the ho... carrying a weapon in her pocket when it was just her phone. Her teachers know Dinah has a large social... and do not want this attitude or behavior to spread to others. This is Dinah's last year in elementary school... year, she will attend the public middle school, which has a more diverse student body and students from all... economic levels.

Tier 2 Elementary School Case #8: <u>Jacob</u>

Kelsey Helgesen, OTR/L

DENT STRENGTHS

ifying personal strengths is critical to promoting hope, increasing self-efficacy, and supporting recovery. To encourage
nued practice with identifying strengths, the editors intentionally provided a blank three-bulleted list for each case. It is
ope that users of the resource will be able to identify even more than three strengths in each vignette.)

CUPATIONAL NEEDS

HOOL BARRIERS: EXTERNALIZING BEHAVIORS

Stealing

Lying and story embellishment

Disruptive behavioral outbursts, including verbal and physical classroom damage

Physically aggressive

Verbal peer conflicts

Tardy

RSONAL FACTOR CONSIDERATIONS

Unstable home environment

History of abuse

Multiple foster care home placements

Older sibling with mental health issues and suicidal ideations

Client Report

Jacob is an 8-year-old third grader at a public elementary school in a high-poverty neighborhood i
York City. He has been at this school since the beginning of the school year, when he moved to a new foster
Jacob's typical school day involves his foster mom driving him to school (he is usually late and picks up a
free breakfast on his way to class), going to class, and being picked up by his foster mom with the other kid
home, including his younger sister. At home, Jacob enjoys playing video games, visiting with his mom tw
month, and playing with his baby sister. At school, he enjoys gym class and working on the computer. Jac
one close friend from his class and has frequent verbal conflicts with other classmates.

Jacob currently lives with his foster mom, her partner, his 2-year-old sister, and two other children in
care. He has been in five foster homes since entering care 2 years ago. He reports that he went into fost
because his mother left him and his baby sister home alone. He also has a 15-year-old sister who is curre
inpatient psychiatric care owing to threatening to kill herself, which Jacob does not talk about and is only
to the school because his foster mother mentioned it to the school assessment team. He speaks positively
his mom after his visits with her at the foster agency.

Jacob does not speak positively about his current foster mom. He reports she curses at him and threa
send him to a new home. He has been abused physically and verbally in previous foster homes. The home
in before his current one he really liked, but he was only there for approximately 1 month when the foster r
told school staff that she was sending him to another home because he stole things whenever they went
store, and therefore, she could not go anywhere with him.

Jacob has difficulty being truthful and often starts telling stories that are very different from his reali
example, when a peer says that he did something fun over the weekend, Jacob will always say that he did tha
thing as well and will elaborate on the story, even when it was clearly untrue. For several weeks, he said that
going home with his mom the next month, but the date he gave passed without him going home, and he ch
his story as though the plan had never been different.

Jacob is generally compliant in class but recently had one large outburst when his teacher took his not
from him. He was very upset that she would not give it back and got so upset that he threw things, curse
knocked a desk over. Since then, he has been aggressive with his teacher more frequently, although he has n
another outburst as severe as that one.

His current foster mother says that he has outbursts at home when he does not get his way and he pu
holes in the wall, although he is not physically aggressive toward other people in the home. She also says that
Jacob is upset, he will curse at her. She wants him to be re-evaluated and placed into a more restrictive s
setting.

Tier 2 Elementary School Case #9: _Sam_

Molly Bathje, PhD, MS, OTR/L

DENT STRENGTHS

*ifying personal strengths is critical to promoting hope, increasing self-efficacy, and supporting recovery. To encourage
nued practice with identifying strengths, the editors intentionally provided a blank three-bulleted list for each case. It is
ope that users of the resource will be able to identify even more than three strengths in each vignette.)*

UPATIONAL NEEDS

HOOL BARRIERS: EXTERNALIZING BEHAVIORS

Intermittent disciplinary problems

Physical aggression with peers

Poor rule compliance

Poor routine transitions

Challenges in following directions with classroom activities

Declining academic performance

Poor emotional regulation, including frequent crying

Negative self-talk

RSONAL FACTOR CONSIDERATIONS

Low self-esteem

Poor sleep routine at home

Older sibling involved with extracurricular activities

Client Report

Sam is 8 years old and in second grade at the local suburban public grammar school. He has one olde
(15 years old) and lives with both his mom and dad. He has lived in the same town and attended the same
since kindergarten. Throughout his school career, he has had intermittent disciplinary problems, mainly
to aggression against other children and not following rules or instructions from his teachers. He also expe
some academic problems owing to not turning in homework and difficulty following instructions on assign
He usually gets along well with peers and has friends, but there have been some instances of aggression and
out when peers disagree with him. Disciplinary issues have recently increased, and his academic performa
been poorer. His parents are interested and engaged in his school performance and have attended meetin
his teacher recently, where they have indicated that he is having emotional mood swings at home with fr
crying and negative self-talk.

Sam's typical school day includes waking up, getting dressed, eating breakfast, completing basic hygien
gathering belonging for school, all encouraged and prompted by his mother. His mother drops him off at
where he joins his classmates in his homeroom after placing his backpack and coat in his cubby area. He a
classes throughout the day, mainly in the same room, but moves with his classmates from his homeroom
lated classes, such as gym, art, recess, and lunch. Transition times are most difficult and when the majority
conflicts occur. After school, he goes to the playground while waiting for his mother to pick him up. After r
ing home, he changes, eats a snack, and watches television, or plays on his tablet for approximately 1 hour. F
dinner with his mother and father and his sister when she is available. She is 15 years old and now particip
multiple after-school clubs and sports activities, which limit her time at home. After dinner, with encourag
from his mother, he does homework for 1 to 1.5 hours, takes a shower, and goes to bed. Bedtime is a cha
he frequently indicates he is not tired and wants to stay up with his tablet or television. Once a week, he a
soccer practice. He wakes up several times on a typical night and goes into his parents' room or his paren
hear him playing in his room. On weekends, Sam and his family are typically busy visiting with family and f
or attending events for him or his sister. They also spend time at home playing in the backyard, going to the
pool, and riding bikes.

Sam reports that he does not like school because there are too many rules, nothing is fun, and he does i
any choice in what they do at school. He says he has friends, but that they do not really like him anymore a
not always include him. He indicates that when he tries to tell the other kids how to do things better, they
listen to him and are mean. He states, "Everyone is always yelling at me" at school. He also indicates that he
smart and he cannot do the hard work the teachers expect him to complete. He indicates that school make
feel bad and he is so happy when the day is over.

Recently, Sam has been more defiant with teachers and is requiring more disciplinary intervention. The
difficult times are during transitions and less structured activities, such as recess and lunch. His academic p
mance is suffering because he is not following directions on in-class assignments and frequently does not ha
homework with him to turn in.

Tier 2 Elementary School Case #10: *Lucas*

Marcela De La Pava, MS, OTR/L
and Laurette Olson, PhD, OTR/L, FAOTA

DENT STRENGTHS

tifying personal strengths is critical to promoting hope, increasing self-efficacy, and supporting recovery. To encourage nued practice with identifying strengths, the editors intentionally provided a blank three-bulleted list for each case. It is ope that users of the resource will be able to identify even more than three strengths in each vignette.)

CUPATIONAL NEEDS

HOOL BARRIERS: EXTERNALIZING BEHAVIORS

Inability to sit still and focus

Difficulty following directions

Impulsivity

Frequently physically overexcited

Difficulty keeping hands to himself

Unable to control his behavior

Disruptive during assemblies, related arts, and other unstructured tasks

Difficulty following classroom rules and routines

Emotional

Social skill immaturity

RSONAL FACTOR CONSIDERATIONS

Affluent family with full-time nanny

Poor emotional regulation

Self-injurious behaviors

Client Report

Lucas is a 5-year-old boy currently attending kindergarten at a public elementary school in a north
U.S. suburb. Lucas lives in a private home with his mother, father, and 2-year-old brother. His parents wo
time in the medical industry and have a live-in nanny who provides full-time child care within their home.
mother is treated for generalized anxiety disorder after two miscarriages before Lucas's birth. Lucas is lovi
affectionate with his parents, younger brother, and other relatives. Although he enjoys playing with his brot
is very particular about sharing his toys and limits what he allows his brother to use.

Lucas loves to draw, paint, and participate in craft activities. He is very creative and loves using his im
tion to tell stories or make up elaborate games. He also likes word searches and puzzles. Playing video ga
also a favored activity, but his parents limit his playtime because Lucas becomes very frustrated when he
successful with a game.

At the parent-teacher conference during the first marking period of the school year, Lucas's kinder
teacher raised concerns regarding his behavior, including "his inability to sit still, focus, and follow direction
stated that Lucas is often disruptive during "specials," such as school assemblies, gym, music, and library, an
less structured times during the school day, such as lunch and recess. He often becomes physically overly
to the point that he cannot control his behavior. He gets too close to other children and has difficulty keep
hands and body to himself.

Lucas's parents reported that Lucas has difficulty interacting with his peers and forming friendship
other children in their neighborhood. Lucas is very outgoing and seeks out other children for play, but then
to be in control of the play situation. For example, if the children decide to play a game, Lucas insists th
children play the game of his choice, play by the rules that he believes are the rules, and then demands that
in charge of how the game proceeds. If things do not go the way that Lucas wants them to go, he gets very
retreats, and refuses to rejoin the play activity with the other children.

Although Lucas wants to go to events like birthday parties to be with other children and make friends
events are particularly challenging for him. A lot of stimulation in an environment is overwhelming to hi
typically starts to cry when there are limits on his ability to play with other children when he has the impu
play. Once Lucas becomes upset, it is very difficult if not "impossible" for him to calm down. Typically, the
leaves the parties early and goes home if Lucas becomes upset because of a seemingly minor limit or rebuf
another child.

His parents describe Lucas as being "very sensitive and very emotional" and that he often exhibits "r
that swing between extremes." According to his mother, Lucas has "extreme" emotional reactions, which s
scribed as "anxiety attacks or panic attacks that can last for what seems like hours." Typically, before Lucas
emotional meltdown, he moves "all over the place," talks about random things that do not make sense, and
he cries and screams. His parents stated that it is very hard to calm him down. His father reports that there
been instances during a meltdown when Lucas has started to slap his (own) face or he may stick his fingers
his mouth until he makes himself gag.

Lucas's parents are very concerned with his social-emotional development. Although Lucas is meetin
demic standards in kindergarten, the parents are worried that his dysregulated behavior and poor social ski
interfere with his ability to do well in school as academic and social demands increase in the first grade. The
want their son to make and keep friends, to be included in social activities, and to enjoy group activities with
children in his class.

Tier 2 Middle School Case #1: _Summer_

Toymika LeFlore, MEd, OTR/L

DENT STRENGTHS

tifying personal strengths is critical to promoting hope, increasing self-efficacy, and supporting recovery. To encourage
nued practice with identifying strengths, the editors intentionally provided a blank three-bulleted list for each case. It is
ope that users of the resource will be able to identify even more than three strengths in each vignette.)

CUPATIONAL NEEDS

HOOL BARRIERS: INTERNALIZING BEHAVIORS

Academic decline from the start of the school year

Limited cooperative task completion

Poor assignment completion

Attention and focus challenges

Absence owing to somatic symptoms and illness

Increasing social isolation owing to peer conflicts

RSONAL FACTOR CONSIDERATIONS

Transitioning to high school next year

Immaturity

Did not make the girls' basketball team

Dropped out of band

Average academic ability; typically an A/B student

Grief and loss with the loss of three extended family deaths

Client Report

Summer is a 13-year-old female student in the eighth grade. She has attended Hyatt Middle School sinc grade. She will be transitioning to high school next school year. Summer is the oldest of four children. She a two-parent home. Both of her parents are employed. Summer's parents desire for her to be more responsi mature. Her mother values education but has an open mind about Summer attending college after high Her parents want her to be happy in whatever career choice she decides to pursue. They have supported everything she participates in.

Summer decided to try out for the girls' basketball team and did not make the team. Summer prev played the clarinet in the school band, and she is a great musician. She no longer has a desire to play the c and has dropped out of the band. Her parents are very disappointed; however, all parties agreed that she to focus on her academic performance first and foremost. The family loves spending time together. Summ a desire to be a chef one day and own multiple restaurants throughout the major cities across the United Her hobbies include cooking for her friends and extended family members and watching cooking shows. Sl enjoys watching YouTube and has boasted of wanting to become a YouTuber by posting videos to earn mo

Summer has struggled academically since the sixth grade. She has the academic ability to complete signments but often just refuses to do so in any of her core classes. She often loses focus in class and be frustrated when redirected by her teachers. She has received multiple office referrals this school year for na ing to nonacademic websites in her classes. She has twice walked out of class and frequently fakes somatic toms to hide out in the nurse's station. She cannot participate in any group projects without having a confli her peers. As a result, Summer's grades are not an accurate reflection of her academic ability. Currently, s all unsatisfactory grades in all core academic classes. A 2.0-grade point average is required to participate eighth-grade activities for all four quarters. Many of her teachers have stayed after school to assist her in in ing her grades. All her teachers reported that she starts the school year very strongly and begins the year fc and motivated to learn; they know she is academically capable. Typically, her grades are all As and Bs durin time. As the quarter comes to an end, her grades begin to decline. She manages to complete and turn in all assignments late for partial credit. This has been enough to maintain a C average.

Summer has reported that middle school has been the most difficult school years for her. She has su the loss of her favorite aunt 2 years ago, and last year, her grandmother and her nanny passed away. She wa close to all of them. Her parents reached out to the school social worker for assistance with Summer copin the grief and loss of her relatives. She participated in a support group at school. In addition, Summer confi her parents that there was too much peer pressure this school year. Students were boasting of having sex, drugs, drinking, and engaging in self-injurious behaviors. She felt like she did not fit in with the kids at her s She was also teased at school for lack of physical development by her male peers. She was able to confide i situation with her math teacher and school social worker.

She and her family are very involved in their church. She felt that those behaviors did not align with wh was being taught at church and at home. Summer does not have many friends at school that she feels she i nected to. Her very close friend from kindergarten transferred to another school in a neighborhood across Visits have been limited since the move.

Tier 2 Middle School Case #2: _Ronnie_

Susan Friuglietti, DHA, MA, OTR/L
and Mark Bumgarner, MS

DENT STRENGTHS

_ifying personal strengths is critical to promoting hope, increasing self-efficacy, and supporting recovery. To encourage
nued practice with identifying strengths, the editors intentionally provided a blank three-bulleted list for each case. It is
ope that users of the resource will be able to identify even more than three strengths in each vignette.)_

CUPATIONAL NEEDS

HOOL BARRIERS: INTERNALIZING BEHAVIORS

Poor academic performance

Avoids social interactions; keeps hoodie up and earbuds in listening to music

Behavior referrals and recent suspension for stealing

Sleeping in class

Refusal to participate in group work

Self-imposed social isolation

Tested into the gifted and talented program; refuses to participate

RSONAL FACTOR CONSIDERATIONS

Biracial

Foster care and a previous failed adoption

Transient living; two to three homes per school year

Parental drug addiction and imprisonment

Poor sleep routine

Low self-esteem

Client Report

Ronnie is a 12-year-old boy in the seventh grade at Summit Rise Middle School in North Carolina biracial and currently in foster care following his mother's drug addiction issues and subsequent overdos Ronnie was 5 years old, leading to his placement in Department of Social Services custody when Ron starting kindergarten. Ronnie's dad was imprisoned for life when Ronnie was 6 months old. When Ron 9 years old, an adoptive placement was located but failed within 1 year owing to Ronnie's significant behavi sues. Ronnie has since moved to his sixth foster home in the past 24 months approximately 1 month ago. R caseworkers have been unstable and that position has often been vacant. His current foster home is a ther placement (White foster mother and Black foster father) that has experience with physical and psycholog sues with foster children. They have expressed an interest in potential adoption if services can be secured him to stabilize and engage in all environments. There are no additional children in the current foster hon Department of Social Services has a legal obligation to provide financial resources for intervention as need Ronnie.

Although Ronnie tested in the gifted category at the end-of-year testing, he is barely passing each with Cs and Ds. Ronnie has changed schools at least two or three times a year owing to the moves in pr foster homes. At school, Ronnie is minimally verbal, avoids social interaction, and does not initiate convers although he responds to direct requests or questions appropriately; at times, however, he keeps his earb his ears whenever he can and he keeps his hoodie up. He loves rap music and enjoys both listening to mus creating his own raps.

Ronnie has had several referrals related to behavioral issues in the classroom, and he was recently susp for stealing a jacket and cash from a student's locker. Ronnie reported that he just wanted the items. Ror often sleeping in class or keeps his head on the desk with his hoodie up. When called on by the teacher, he minimal responses and says anything asked of him is "stupid." When asked to keep his head upright and pay tion, he keeps an upright posture but keeps his earbuds in. On two occasions, he has refused to engage when to participate in a group activity during class, walked out of the room, and did not return. The only teach reports that Ronnie pays attention in class is his music teacher, who says that Ronnie pays close attention lessons on music structure and the history of music and that his assignments in music class have been insi and demonstrate a talent for music.

Although Ronnie has not made any friends at his new school yet, he does talk superficially to the two foster children that are currently at the middle school. When asked, Ronnie reports the other students look at him for not being normal, and it is not worth getting to know them anyway because he does not know hov he will be at the school.

Ronnie does say his new foster home is OK and his foster mom cooks well. He also likes that he is th child at the house and he has his own room for the first time and can listen to music in his room. Ronnie p to stay in his room; however, he is now willing to perform chores as requested and has occasionally indepen initiated washing the dishes after dinner. He thinks his foster dad is cool because he has come in and lister his music with him and has offered to teach him how to play the guitar. Ronnie would like to find a perm home and not keep moving.

Tier 2 Middle School Case #3: *Yael*

Paula Cook, OTD, OTR/L
and Ashley Fecht, OTD, OTR/L, BCP

STUDENT STRENGTHS

(Identifying personal strengths is critical to promoting hope, increasing self-efficacy, and supporting recovery. To encourage continued practice with identifying strengths, the editors intentionally provided a blank three-bulleted list for each case. It is our hope that users of the resource will be able to identify even more than three strengths in each vignette.)

OCCUPATIONAL NEEDS

SCHOOL BARRIERS: INTERNALIZING BEHAVIORS

Late and incomplete assignments

Limited social interactions and no identified friendships

Academic concerns in English language arts

Easily distracted with poor attention

Self-imposed isolation from school-related activities and events

PERSONAL FACTOR CONSIDERATIONS

Anxiety

Embarrassment and shame

Juvenile rheumatoid arthritis with consequent extremity limitations impacting gait and hand use

Father is often gone from the home owing to his job as a pilot

Prefers adult companionship

Low self-esteem

Client Report

Yael is a seventh-grade student at Spring Mountain Academy, a charter elementary school in Las Nevada. She is 13 years old and was diagnosed with juvenile rheumatoid arthritis at age 11 years. Her olde who is 17 years old, attends the local public high school. Her father is a commercial airline pilot and often g trips for several days up to a week at a time. Yael's mom is an attorney.

A typical day for Yael includes her mother driving her and her sister to school every day. Yael is drop first and arrives about 20 minutes before the first bell. This allows her to get to her locker early and get before the hallways are too crowded. She is pulled out of the English language block for reading suppo has previously received occupational therapy for written communication and to maximize school partici opportunities. She has appropriate assistive technology and accommodations to allow her to be successf academic expectations.

When asked about her friends, Yael says that her sister is her best friend and has trouble identifying st in her class as her friends. This is consistent with teacher observations. Other students in her class are p her but do not connect with her as a friend and keep their distance from her. Teachers and staff at the sch endeared by Yael and concerned that she seems to prefer their company over that of other students. Yael she had a friend or two at school or at least someone who knows her well.

Yael's favorite class is music. Her second favorite class is math. She dislikes English and writing but enjo tening to audiobooks. She enjoys chorus and would like to audition for the performing chorus but is afraid s not be successful. For a cultural awareness day at school, she brought in some of her mother's homemade rug and the other students refused to try it. The staff, however, loved it. Yael enjoys baking with her mother and She also likes painting her nails, her sparkly shoes, listening to music, and playing the piano.

Yael has had some anxiety over her juvenile rheumatoid arthritis now that she is in middle school. Thi ety over appearance has led her to focus on her outward appearance. She has begun wearing makeup, whi applies at school, and she is trying to lose weight. The lunchroom monitor has observed her throwing aw lunches. Her teacher noticed that Yael seems more distracted than usual. She is hiding her significant weig by wearing baggy clothes. Her mom and sister noticed that Yael now spends more time alone in her roo stares at herself in every reflective surface she passes. Yael has avoided all school events this year, and her attributed it to her being embarrassed about her juvenile rheumatoid arthritis and did not want to force he

Tier 2 Middle School Case #4: *Jason*

Bobbi Carrlson, PhD, OTR/L; Sarah Nielsen, PhD, OTR/L, FAOTA; and Janet S. Jedlicka, PhD, OTR/L, FAOTA

‏DENT STRENGTHS

‏tifying personal strengths is critical to promoting hope, increasing self-efficacy, and supporting recovery. To encourage ‏nued practice with identifying strengths, the editors intentionally provided a blank three-bulleted list for each case. It is ‏ope that users of the resource will be able to identify even more than three strengths in each vignette.)

‏CUPATIONAL NEEDS

‏HOOL BARRIERS: EXTERNALIZING BEHAVIORS

Poor academic performance

Executive dysfunction impacting organization, multistep assignments, time management, task initiation, and task completion

Poor emotional regulation

Refusal to participate in challenging assignments

Argues and verbally yells and screams at classroom teachers and peers

Immaturity

Refuses to participate in group work

Impulsivity

No identified close social relationships

‏RSONAL FACTOR CONSIDERATIONS

Feels stupid and embarrassed

Lacks age-appropriate process skills

Lives with mother, stepfather, and infant baby brother

Sees his dad once per month and when they play video games online together

Client Report

Jason is a 12-year-old boy who is a sixth grader at Washington Middle School. This is his second year school. He transferred to Washington Middle School midway in fifth grade when his stepfather was transfe his employer. Washington Middle School consists of grades 5 through 8 with four sections in each grade. St begin to transition between all core classes in sixth grade in addition to related arts, including physical edu and music. He rides the bus to school, which arrives just before the start of his 8:20 AM class, and particip after-school athletics until 5 PM when his stepdad picks him up. His teachers have been concerned with his to organize his materials for classes and complete increasingly complex assignments at his grade level. The ers also indicated Jason has difficulty regulating his emotions during these times. Jason was recently dia; with ADHD and executive dysfunction.

Jason currently lives in an apartment with his infant brother, mom, and stepdad. He sees his birth d proximately one time per month but speaks to him multiple times per week when gaming. His mother repo met most of his motor milestones but scooted on his bottom instead of creeping on his hands. He was not creep until after he began walking. Mom stated that with the new baby at home it has been more difficult to make sure Jason has completed all of his work correctly and has placed it into his backpack. Mom reporte Jason becomes upset when asked to stop playing his video games or is reminded to finish his chores. He freq needs reminders to finish all parts of his chores at home, such as replacing a garbage bag when taking the g out or loading all the dishes into the dishwasher. During these times, he goes to his room and refuses to con She would like him to be more independent with his homework and chores.

Jason struggles to complete multistep assignments during his school day and for homework. He freq misses portions of his assignments, both with in-class activities and homework. When corrected or a mis pointed out by a peer or teacher, Jason becomes upset, argues, and states that he "hates the sixth grade ar wants to go home." He then sits in a desk with his arms crossed and refuses to participate in his academ the remainder of the class period. Jason's peers have begun to show frustration when they are paired wit for activities in class. Jason stated that he likes to be with his peers but feels bad when they do not want to with him. Jason loves to draw and paint; however, he does this freestyle and does not follow directions or a i He used to love building LEGO blocks, but became frustrated when he could not complete complex desigi now does not play with them. His favorite activity is playing video games online with his birth dad, who l a different state.

Jason is active in after-school sports during all seasons but feels he is not good at them and would rather his time playing video games or drawing. He stated that he would like to do well in school but feels stupid wl does poorly on his work, so he does not want to go. Jason also wants to be liked by his peers but gets embari when they do not want to work with him, so he does not want to try.

Tier 2 Middle School Case #5: *Jeremiah*

Karen Stornello, OTD, OTR/L
and Renee Harris, COTA/L

DENT STRENGTHS

tifying personal strengths is critical to promoting hope, increasing self-efficacy, and supporting recovery. To encourage nued practice with identifying strengths, the editors intentionally provided a blank three-bulleted list for each case. It is ope that users of the resource will be able to identify even more than three strengths in each vignette.)

CUPATIONAL NEEDS

HOOL BARRIERS: EXTERNALIZING BEHAVIORS

Frequent school absences

Concerns with physical aggression toward teachers and peers

Academic deficits

Impulsive and makes careless academic mistakes

Multiple behavior referrals for bullying smaller and younger students

RSONAL FACTOR CONSIDERATIONS

Significant social history that includes neglect, trauma, and abuse

Takes medication for disrupted mood disorder

Unstable living environment

No identified future goals

Client Report

Jeremiah is 12 years old and a sixth-grade student. He was hospitalized in 2016, diagnosed with ADHI traumatic stress disorder, and disruptive mood regulation disorder. He began taking a mood-stabilizing n tion at that time. Upon returning to school after the hospitalization, he hit the principal and social worker. this event, Jeremiah's significant social history was discovered. He lived in Florida with his grandfather fo years. While there, his aunt and his sister cared for him. He moved from house to house as different family bers were able to care for him at different times. He has a history of family violence, including his uncle set on fire resulting in his death, which Jeremiah witnessed. The Department of Social Services was prev involved owing to neglect, including lack of food. There are also reports of physical abuse when he was livir a stepfather. His mother and father have a history of being incarcerated.

Jeremiah reports that he worries about his mother because she has been in and out of prison, and he ha with her intermittently through the years. He currently lives with a godmother. He reportedly gets alon his godmother but fights with his sister—yelling, swearing, hitting, and kicking her. His godmother repor Jeremiah's home life is chaotic, with a history of fighting and violence.

In a psychological report from January 2017, Jeremiah was below average in word reading and very math problem-solving and numerical operations. Overall, Jeremiah's disjointed childhood has affected his s in school. In the past 2 school years, he has had frequent absences owing to his unstable living environme is typically healthy.

His daily school routine consists of taking private transportation to school and attending classes 7:45 AM until 3:00 PM. School provides breakfast and lunch for all students. He participates in differe math, reading, and language arts, and daily social-emotional learning activities (personal development), s social studies, daily physical education, and art once a week. Jeremiah has had multiple behavioral referra are often the result of impulsive thinking and actions. He is known to consistently bully several children w smaller and younger. Jeremiah is motivated to work for daily rewards but is unable to identify goals for the

Tier 2 Middle School Case #6: *Richie*

Gina Rainelli, OTD, OTR/L

DENT STRENGTHS

*tifying personal strengths is critical to promoting hope, increasing self-efficacy, and supporting recovery. To encourage
nued practice with identifying strengths, the editors intentionally provided a blank three-bulleted list for each case. It is
ope that users of the resource will be able to identify even more than three strengths in each vignette.)*

CUPATIONAL NEEDS

HOOL BARRIERS: EXTERNALIZING BEHAVIORS

Academic deficits

Impulsive violent behavioral responses, including throwing chairs and yelling

Poor cooperative behavior skills

Challenges with unstructured school events, including lunch and after school

RSONAL FACTOR CONSIDERATIONS

Significant social history that includes neglect

Oppositional defiant disorder and ADHD

Lives with maternal grandmother and older sister

Sensitive to environmental stimuli

Client Report

Richie is a 14-year-old eighth-grade student. He currently attends Westland Middle School in an urban district. He has attended Westland Middle School for 3 months. Richie has previously been suspended at school for kicking, use of curse words, running from class and the school building, and making weapon classroom materials. He currently lives with his grandma and an older sister. His mom and his stepfather prison for drug-related crimes. When Richie's mom was pregnant with him, her husband attacked and be causing early labor. Richie was born at 35 weeks, and his twin did not survive. His biological father is also in for that offense. Richie has lived with his grandmother since he was 6 years old, when Child Protective S took him and his sister from his parents owing to neglect. Richie has a diagnosis of oppositional defiant di and ADHD. He does not take medication currently.

Richie reports that he likes his current school because he likes his teacher. He is below grade level in ing and math and this frustrates him, although he says he is "getting it more" than when he was at his last Richie's favorite class is physical education, but he likes science too. He reports he has one friend but not at because they are mean to him at school. Richie says he likes the teachers he has because they help him an him points toward rewards when he gets his work done. Richie said he wants to be a truck driver when he up or maybe a baker, but he has not decided yet. Richie believes that he is smart and is improving in readi math every day, but he still needs help.

His teacher describes him as a "really neat kid," expressing that he loves nature, bugs, and butterflies and interested in science. His teacher also says he gets upset when it is too loud or when people accidentally touc He may yell or swear or hit another student if they get too close to him. Richie has difficulty cooperating and ing out with other students during lunch and unstructured school events. It was reported that he responds a calm adult who can explain to him what happened, why, and what he can do instead. He has been restrain times in the last month for out-of-control physical behavior (throwing a chair in the classroom).

At home, Richie stays inside and plays video games or watches television by himself because his sister ally with friends in her room and his grandma works. His grandma will not let him play outside alone becau neighborhood is not safe. Richie goes to church every Sunday with his grandma and spends time with his uncles, and cousins after church.

Tier 2 High School Case #1: *Zoey*

Teri K. Rupp, MOT, OTR/L, C/NDT
and Patricia Bowyer, EdD, MS, OTR, FAOTA, SFHEA

DENT STRENGTHS

tifying personal strengths is critical to promoting hope, increasing self-efficacy, and supporting recovery. To encourage nued practice with identifying strengths, the editors intentionally provided a blank three-bulleted list for each case. It is ope that users of the resource will be able to identify even more than three strengths in each vignette.)

CUPATIONAL NEEDS

HOOL BARRIERS: EXTERNALIZING BEHAVIORS

History of discipline referrals

Intermittent social isolation

Physical peer altercations

Disrespectful behavior toward adult staff

Recent suspension

Frequent absence from classes

RSONAL FACTOR CONSIDERATIONS

Foster care home environment

Depression and anxiety

Inconsistent home environment

Drug use

No healthy coping skills

Client Report

Zoey is a 16-year-old junior attending Franklin High School. This school year is her first year att
Franklin. Zoey was removed from her last foster home after her foster family discovered inappropriate ph
her on her foster brother's cell phone. She has denied sending the photos to him or engaging in any sexual
ior. She has been with her new foster family, the Walkers, for 6 months. Her new foster parents work in the
district as a bus driver and a teacher. Her medical records indicate diagnoses of ADHD, depression, anxie
possible autism spectrum disorder. She has a history of discipline referrals and challenges throughout her
career relating to her depression and anxiety. She recently received a psychiatric evaluation owing to aggres
her foster home and suicidal thoughts.

Zoey's typical school routine begins with her riding the school bus and socializing with students in th
mon area before school starts at 7:45 AM. She attends classes in core subjects, eats lunch alone while re
and returns home on the bus at 3:30 PM. She has shown behavioral challenges during the transition to h
school and foster home, including physical altercations with other students and disrespectful behavior t
staff. Recently, this behavior has increased, and she has had three physical altercations with other students
last 90 days, resulting in a total of 6 days of suspension. Since her last suspension, she has been skipping clas
fusing to engage in school work during class, and having verbal outbursts when redirected by staff membe
behavioral overreactions toward staff have escalated into her eloping from school. She is currently failing f
her six classes owing to her refusal to complete work, her skipping core classes, and her behavioral outburs
case manager and foster parents are concerned she will fail the 11th grade and drop out of school. She is sche
to age out of the foster care system in 2 years when she turns 18.

Zoey reported that she does not see a reason to go to school and does not see herself going to college or l
a career. She said, "Girls like me have no one and go nowhere." She was unable to articulate any goals for her
other than finding a boyfriend. She says that a boy in her previous foster home loved her, but that her c
foster family will not allow her to see him. She has been texting him, and he has not responded or shown up
they have agreed to meet, but she knows he loves her. When referring to the fights with other students, sh
that they deserved it because they called her a liar, tried to steal her personal belongings from her desk, and
not listen to her when she was talking to them in the hallway. She feels her teachers are stupid and she a
did work being assigned in her previous school. She knows the information and will never use it, so "why s
I attend class or complete work I already know and won't ever need?" Her teachers reported that she is high
ticulate and will lie about completing work, where she has been, or what she is doing. Zoey often convinces s
giving her a break and is rarely held accountable for her behavior. She reports feeling anxious about "life" an
"stuck" and "alone." Zoey knows that she has "big feelings" and has trouble controlling these when she is ang
frustrated. Zoey was recently found to be using crack cocaine and meth.

Zoey feels very unsure about where she will be living from year to year and hates that she does not have
thing that belongs to her. Zoey feels she does not have a history or important personal milestones like othe
and does not have any healthy coping skills. She will be aging out of the foster care system soon and worries
what will happen and where she will go. Zoey knows that a high school diploma will be essential to her
after age 18 years, but does not feel she will graduate owing to her unstable living situations and being a fost

Zoey engages in mostly solitary activities, such as reading or social media. She reports having close frien
the internet in her online gaming community, but she has never met them. She uses the computer to learn h
do many things that no one will teach her in her foster homes, like fashion and makeup. She says she enjo
social activities at school, but "I do not have friends and feel lonely when I go to school clubs or activities."
responsible for making dinner once a week, cleaning her room, and washing her clothes, but she takes a long
to complete these chores without an adult reminding her and staying on her until the job is complete. She
not feel that she belongs or fits in at school or in her foster family because she is so different from them and
not have a life story or connections with people and places like her peers.

Tier 2 High School Case #2: _Ben_

Andrea Thinnes, OTD, OTR/L, FNAP
and Anna Domina, OTD, OTR/L

DENT STRENGTHS

tifying personal strengths is critical to promoting hope, increasing self-efficacy, and supporting recovery. To encourage nued practice with identifying strengths, the editors intentionally provided a blank three-bulleted list for each case. It is ope that users of the resource will be able to identify even more than three strengths in each vignette.)

CUPATIONAL NEEDS

HOOL BARRIERS: INTERNALIZING BEHAVIORS

Sleeping in class

Academic delay in English language arts

Social isolation

Limited participation in school functions

RSONAL FACTOR CONSIDERATIONS

Father in the military → currently deployed

Adopted sibling and an older brother who is a star football player at the high school

Parent performance pressure

Anxiety

Gay; not known to others

Client Report

Ben is a 14-year-old freshman at Mayville High School. He lives at home with his mother, father, a
siblings. His mother is a stay-at-home mom, and his father is active military and has been deployed for 3
now. Ben has an older brother, Charlie, who is a senior at the same high school and a star football player.
has a younger sister, Claire, who is in first grade at the local elementary school. Claire was adopted from
when she was 5 years old.

Ben's daily routine consists of getting up early to ride to school with his brother who has weight lifting
class each morning. Ben is usually found in the mornings with another male student named Tony, who a
rives at school early for tutoring. He tends to skip his tutoring session, so he can go out back of the cafet
smoke. Tony and Ben bonded over their mutual struggle with classes and the pressure they feel to perfor
ter in school from their parents. They find a common interest in spending time alone or with a limited gr
friends. Ben waits until the last minute to arrive at his first period class, English, which is a subject he ha
having difficulty keeping up with notes and reading. As the day progresses, Ben is usually found sleeping i
In the evenings, Ben prefers to watch television alone and falls asleep on the couch most days. This behavi
escalated since his dad was deployed, and he is feeling more anxious than normal. Ben has known he was
several years but has not come out to his family, and he does not believe anyone at the high school knows.

Ben has had numerous office referrals owing to sleeping in class, and this has resulted in his mother
called in for a meeting owing to the high volume in only the first quarter of the school year. Ben was diag
with dyslexia in the sixth grade but has had minimal intervention in the school setting. His grades and test
have been slipping since starting high school.

Ben describes himself as a loyal person to his family, friends, and country. He prefers to keep to himse
is more introverted and not athletic. Ben would say that he is a good percussion player and enjoys writing
He has a small group of friends that like to get together for a jam session after school. He also says that schoo
not interest him and that the things the teachers expect are just not important or too hard.

Ben is very independent. He spends time on his own at home because Charlie is usually gone at practic
games or out with friends and his mother is busy with Claire, who has been struggling with assimilation sin
adoption. Ben has developed an interest in cooking, especially Italian food because his new friend, Tony, is

Tier 2 High School Case #3: *Jack*

Allen Keener, OTD, MS, OTR/L, ATP

DENT STRENGTHS

ifying personal strengths is critical to promoting hope, increasing self-efficacy, and supporting recovery. To encourage nued practice with identifying strengths, the editors intentionally provided a blank three-bulleted list for each case. It is ope that users of the resource will be able to identify even more than three strengths in each vignette.)

CUPATIONAL NEEDS

HOOL BARRIERS: INTERNALIZING AND EXTERNALIZING BEHAVIORS

Late to class

Social isolation

Sleeping in class

Stealing

Declining academic performance; missed assignments

RSONAL FACTOR CONSIDERATIONS

New town and new school

No family or friend support

Poverty

Hunger

Caring for younger brother

Overwhelmed with family responsibilities

Client Report

Jack is a 13-year-old student at Morgantown High School, which is located in a midsize city. Jack ide
with the pronouns they/them. This is their first year in the school district due to their mom moving the fa
this new city in order to pursue a better-paying job. Jack lives in a small apartment with their mother an
5-year-old brother. They do not have any family or friends in this new location.

Jack's mom has been working two jobs to provide for them and the younger brother, who attends an el
tary school on the other side of town. Jack is often late for class because they are expected to accompan
brother to school, then they have to walk to Morgantown High. Jack frequently does not have lunch or
money in their school lunch account or the needed supplies for class. They reported to the lunchroom work
one teacher that their mom told Jack that money was tight. Because there is no public transportation availat
needed money for gas for her commute, and that took priority over school supplies and books.

Usually, Jack sits alone and has not been observed interacting with any classmates. They do not appear t
many friends but are pleasant and respectful to others. Recently, Jack has been falling asleep during class a
caught trying to steal two bags of potato chips in the busy lunchroom. While investigating the incident, te
reported a change in attitude, disorganization, and Jack lashing out to the counselor who was collecting
mation. One teacher indicated that Jack seems to be carrying the "weight of the world" on their shoulder
has not submitted a homework assignment in a few weeks now, and when confronted, they just shrugge
shoulders. Jack's grades are falling, and they appear to be even more withdrawn in class. One of Jack's te
attempted to contact Jack's mother to discuss her concerns, but the telephone number was not in service. S
officials agree that some action is needed, but there is not a consensus regarding the most appropriate appr

After class, when asked about an assignment they had not turned in, Jack told the math teacher that hom
was not important to them because Jack had to care for their brother every day. Jack told the teacher the
so much to do in one day and it was overwhelming to try to do everything they are supposed to do. Susp
more might be going on, Jack was referred to the guidance counselor. The counselor offered them a snack,
Jack devoured, stating that they had not eaten breakfast. When asked why, Jack stated they spend their mo
making sure their brother is ready for school because it is their responsibility. Jack revealed their mother is
ing long hours at multiple jobs and Jack and their brother are alone most of the time. Jack stated to the cou
they feel they have to be a parent even though Jack is only 13 years old, and that it is difficult to be worried
school when there is so much responsibility at home.

As the session continues, the counselor learns that Jack is shouldering the majority of the household c
care of the brother, and making simple meals for them to eat. During the conversation, Jack begins to cry an
the counselor there is too much going on in their life. Jack states, "I just want to be a regular kid, but I don't
how. I want to have friends and do things that I want to do."

Tier 2 High School Case #4: *Sarah*

Ryan Thomure, OTD, OTR/L, LCSW
and Ray Cendejas, COTA/L

DENT STRENGTHS

*tifying personal strengths is critical to promoting hope, increasing self-efficacy, and supporting recovery. To encourage
nued practice with identifying strengths, the editors intentionally provided a blank three-bulleted list for each case. It is
ope that users of the resource will be able to identify even more than three strengths in each vignette.)*

CUPATIONAL NEEDS

HOOL BARRIERS: INTERNALIZING AND EXTERNALIZING BEHAVIORS

Declining academic performance

Inconsistent completion of school assignments

Distracted in class

Decreased success with school and home roles and responsibilities

Time management

RSONAL FACTOR CONSIDERATIONS

Long train commute to school

Stress

Difficulty with organizational skills and planning

Poor success with balancing responsibilities and preferred activities

Client Report

Sarah, age 17 years, is a junior at Joel Miller Memorial High School. Sarah's school is located in a resi[...] neighborhood within a large, urban city. Sarah has lived in an urban environment for most of her life[...] comfortable with most aspects of city life, such as use of public transportation, culture, and safety. Sarah is [...] teenager whose typical daily routine involves taking the train to and from school, attending class, participa[...] her school's debate club, and playing video games and music with friends. Additionally, Sarah has a boyfrien[...] she has been dating for 4 months. Sarah has been a strong student for most of her time in school but has re[...] begun receiving Cs and Ds and has even failed several assignments. She has become inconsistent in comple[...] homework assignments, and her parents report that she has not seemed as engaged at home.

In a meeting regarding her struggles in school, Sarah reported that she knows she is struggling in [...] and cannot identify why. She reports that her stress levels have been elevated of late and she has had a har[...] "thinking clearly." She said that sometimes she has trouble keeping track of which assignments are due w[...] which social activity she has committed to on a given night or weekend.

Sarah shared that she highly values the activities she is currently involved in—debate club, a band with fr[...] a new boyfriend, and other activities, like hanging out with friends and spending time with her new boy[...] She reports that she and her friends formed her band, Sarah and the Fireflies, at the start of this school ye[...] they practice one to two times per week in most weeks. The debate club meets once per week, she tries to s[...] boyfriend at least once per week, and she plays video games with friends one to two times per week, in ad[...] to other responsibilities at home, such as household chores and occasionally babysitting her little sister wh[...] parents work late or go to the theater.

Sarah reports that she perceives her commute to and from school to be a significant barrier. Sarah go[...] magnet school outside of her neighborhood and typically has to be on public transportation for 45 min[...] 1 hour each way to get to and from school. Sarah reports that she most often spends that time "zoning out."

Sarah reports that she has a "normal" home life at home with her mother, father, and younger sister. [...] basic needs are met at home, and she participates in typical household chores, such as washing the dishes, m[...] the lawn, and walking the family dog, Franklin. Sarah's parents report that in addition to her recent struggle[...] grades and homework, Sarah has been less attentive to tasks at home and that Franklin has often had to wh[...] walks when Sarah would previously take him out more regularly. Sarah reluctantly admitted these lapses at [...] in conversations with school staff and her parents.

After extensive discussion, school staff, Sarah, and her parents agreed that Sarah is having a challengin[...] balancing the various responsibilities in her life. Sarah does not want to scale back any of her newer activitie[...] her band and boyfriend, but admits she is having trouble managing all the things going on in her life at th[...] ment. Sarah and her parents agree that she needs to develop a more sustainable routine, improve role balanc[...] attempt to decrease continued struggles at school and at home.

Tier 2 High School Case #5: *Cathy*

Linda M. Olson, PhD, OTR/L, FAOTA

DENT STRENGTHS

tifying personal strengths is critical to promoting hope, increasing self-efficacy, and supporting recovery. To encourage nued practice with identifying strengths, the editors intentionally provided a blank three-bulleted list for each case. It is ope that users of the resource will be able to identify even more than three strengths in each vignette.)

CUPATIONAL NEEDS

HOOL BARRIERS: INTERNALIZING AND EXTERNALIZING BEHAVIORS

School performance is declining

Increased social isolation

Increased distractibility

Reports feelings of being overwhelmed to school guidance counselor

RSONAL FACTOR CONSIDERATIONS

Intact traditional family with mom, dad, and younger brother

Mom is diagnosed with breast cancer, which has increased role responsibilities at home for Cathy and her younger brother

High anxiety

Easily overstimulated and overwhelmed

Overwhelmed with family responsibilities

Client Report

Cathy is a 16-year-old junior at Mt. Pleasant High School, in Mt. Pleasant, Illinois, a suburb of Chicag is the suburb where Cathy grew up and has gone through the public school system in Mt. Pleasant with th group of friends since kindergarten. Cathy's daily routine includes having her mom take her to and from attending class, and participating in band practice after school. When she gets home from school, she has helps her mom clean up after dinner, completes her homework, and goes to bed at approximately 9:30 PM. has always been a good student, stating she really enjoys school. She is planning to study economics afte school and is hoping to attend the University of Chicago.

Cathy reports she appreciates the structure that the school year routine brings, stating it helps with f of personal causation and overall productivity. She states she feels lost during the summer and is not sure structure her time. As a result of the decreased structure, she feels guilty that she is not as productive as she she should be because she is not accomplishing daily goals. This in turn results in increased feelings of anxie ther decreasing engagement in productive activities for fear of not being useful or "enough." Cathy's appre for structure is also noted in her daily chores and when she is asked to run errands for her mother. If she is as go to a store or complete a task that she is not familiar with, she becomes highly anxious, which greatly int with her completing the required task; a decrease in accuracy is also noted, which further increases her an

Cathy's interests are limited and tend to be more solitary. Although she plays drums in marching and c bands, she states she does not really enjoy it. She states she enjoys the concert band more because it is easier cus on the music. She states that in the marching band she becomes overstimulated and distracted with eve moving around trying to complete the weekly routine. She also reports increased anxiety when the band di makes last minute changes to the marching band routine. Her other interests include reading, playing con games, completing logic puzzles, and watching television.

Cathy has many acquaintances through school but reports only a few close friends that she hangs ou outside of school. She lives at home with her mother, father, and younger brother. Her dad is an accountan a major accounting firm. Her mother is a stay-at-home mom who has always been involved in helping wi children's school activities as needed. Cathy reports a loving and supportive family.

Cathy's mother was recently diagnosed with breast cancer. She has had surgery and is currently unden chemotherapy. This has made her mother sick, and combined with the limitations after surgery, interfere her ability to engage in instrumental activities of daily living. As a result, Cathy and her brother have been to help with completing these instrumental activities of daily living. Cathy has been asked to oversee the preparation, including shopping for groceries. Her mother does her best to sit down with Cathy to prej weekly menu and grocery list but is not always able to complete this task, leaving Cathy to complete the ta addition to her mother being sick, Cathy's sudden increase in household responsibilities, including meal pla and shopping, has rocked her personal causation and increased her anxiety to the point that she has experi several panic attacks in the grocery store. Over the past few weeks, she has forgotten to purchase things c shopping list, as well as left the store without getting her change and/or not getting the correct amount of ch

Since Cathy has taken on these extra responsibilities, her teachers and friends have noticed a change i at school. Her school performance is slipping, she seems to be more distracted, and has been more withd While meeting with her advisor, Cathy became tearful, stating, "I just can't do this. I don't know how to tak of the house. I was never responsible for grocery shopping. I don't know what I'm doing! Everyone is expe too much of me!"

Tier 2 High School Case #6: *Hailee*

*Aubrey Sejuit, PhD, LISW-CP, LCAS, MEd, GCDF
and Jerry Dye, Jr., MA, MEd, NCC, LCMHCA-NC*

DENT STRENGTHS

*tifying personal strengths is critical to promoting hope, increasing self-efficacy, and supporting recovery. To encourage
nued practice with identifying strengths, the editors intentionally provided a blank three-bulleted list for each case. It is
ope that users of the resource will be able to identify even more than three strengths in each vignette.)*

CUPATIONAL NEEDS

HOOL BARRIERS: INTERNALIZING AND EXTERNALIZING BEHAVIORS

Late and missing school assignments and responsibilities

Declining peer relationships

Declining academic performance

High school transition plan upended

RSONAL FACTOR CONSIDERATIONS

College application denial

Poor self-esteem

Feeling defeated and rejected

Worry about parental disappointment

Client Report

Hailee, age 17 years, is a senior at Shamokin Area Junior/Senior High School, in a town where she ha
since birth. Hailee comes from a close-knit family. Hailee's typical daily school routine involves driving to
with her best friend, attending class, and color guard practice after school. Class sizes are average, and Haile
in a safe, low-crime town with many opportunities for extracurricular and philanthropic involvement. Alt
safe, Hailee's town is composed of lower socioeconomic factors that affect high school graduation rates. H
school has one of the highest dropout rates in the state. An average student, Hailee has been struggling with
ing her friends all get accepted early admission to Penn State University, Syracuse University, and the Uni
of South Carolina. Hailee was recently denied from what she deemed her safety school, and she is contem
going active duty in the military after taking the Armed Services Vocational Aptitude Battery instead of her
plan to become a reservist because she fears she will not get into a college of her choice. She scored high e
on the Armed Services Vocational Aptitude Battery to enlist as an intelligence analyst, like her favorite aunt.
point, she thought about joining the U.S. Army Reserves to help her pay for college, but after being denied
one of seven schools she applied to, Hailee is feeling defeated and is no longer interested in college.

Hailee's mood has been irritable and she has a decreased self-esteem. Hailee had dreams of becoming a
worker and earning her bachelor's degree in social work, but after she was denied from one school, her
quickly faded. She no longer seems interested in keeping up her grades or being as active in extracurricular
ties. Hailee has been handing in homework late and skipping color guard practice.

Hailee has also stopped driving to school with her best friend and instead now takes the school bus.
viewed as extroverted, Hailee no longer follows her friends on social media or responds to text messages
them. When asked about her lack of involvement, she replied, "What's the point? I was already denied. I
need college. I'm sick of going to practice to be around all my friends who know what they are doing with
lives because they got into college and I can't even get into my safety school." She is indecisive about her
and feels hopeless. If Hailee continues to skip color guard practice, she will be kicked out of the high school
Attempting to avoid her friends has started to place a strain on her relationships with them. Handing in l
work late is also beginning to affect her grades in class, which in turn, may affect the possibility of graduating
school. Even if Hailee decides not to attend college, the army recruiter explained that she would need to gra
with her high school diploma to enlist.

Hailee reported that she does not like going to practice anymore. It has become uncomfortable for her
around her friends Hadley, Harper, and Lindsey after they were all accepted to their dream schools. Gen
Hailee enjoys being around people and getting involved in her community. Hailee's uncle, Matt, is an Ope
Iraqi Freedom veteran who served with the 1st battalion and 2nd Marines as a corpsman, and her great gra
ther is a Vietnam War veteran. Because of this, Hailee has a strong desire to serve her country and support
nizations that affect veterans. Her aunt is a member of the junior league and an active alumna in her sorori
Mu, so Hailee enjoys helping raise money for philanthropic causes, such as Children's Miracle Network Hos
and THON. She has helped to raise money for the Stephen Siller Tunnel to Towers 5K, Friends of Fisher F
and Mental Illness Recovery Center, Inc. Hailee also raised money to walk for the National Alliance on M
Illness because mental illness runs in her family, and she was diagnosed with persistent depressive disorder
thymia) last school year. Overall, Hailee enjoys giving back to her community, and until recently, wanted to a
college and join her aunt's sorority.

Although Hailee's counselor provided her with psychoeducation on her diagnosis, she is struggling to p
mental health first. Hailee is feeling disappointed in herself and has increased anxiety and uncertainty abo
future. She is feeling pressured to make her family proud and beginning to question some of her life choices. A
time of this assessment, Hailee was dressed appropriately and appeared neat and well-groomed; her affect se
to be normal. She denied suicidal ideation or plan.

Section 1

...lee describes herself as usually ambitious, happy, and smart. Hailee is described by her family and teachers ...igent, talkative, assertive, and caring. Her school counselor noted that these are the qualities she helped ...o see would be beneficial in the social work field. Hailee's friends describe her as a leader and loyal. ...hout her time at Shamokin Area, Hailee has been on the honor roll and won various awards. In the sum-...ailee has attended the Make a Difference leadership program. Hailee also serves as the public relations ...the Students Against Destructive Decisions, and she is president of the Environmental Club. Hailee still ...her middle school teacher, Mrs. Ramage, who has supported her desire to become a social worker and join ...tary; her favorite high school teacher, Mr. Marcinek, has supported her desire to attend college and join a ...because he was a member of a fraternity at Susquehanna University. She has a strong network of people ...ect her life in a positive way.

...lee describes her home life as typical and satisfying. Her parents love her, and she has a good relationship ...r younger brother. She believes her parents are in a loving relationship, and they all travel as a family dur-...summers when Hailee returns from her leadership program. Hailee's mother stays at home, but earned ...y childhood education degree from the local university, and her father is in construction. She has a long ...relatives who served in the military, and her family is very patriotic. Hailee knows that, without joining the ...y, she may be unable to afford college. Although her father did not attend college, Hailee is aware that her ...value education. Although Hailee is feeling disappointed because she was denied from one college already, ...l wants to make her family proud.

Section 2

Screening and Assessment Tools

Egan, B. E., Sears, C., & Keener, A. (Eds.). *Occupational Therapy Groups for*
Mental Health Challenges in School-Aged Populations: A Tier 2 Resource (p

The No Child Left Behind Public Law 107-110 was signed by former President George W. Bush on J 8, 2002, and created significant changes throughout the national education system. One significant highl No Child Left Behind was the mandate for stronger accountability measures, which increased the importa assessment and data collection to reflect and monitor results.

Using assessment measures to guide evidence-based practice are expectations of occupational therap titioners as reflected in the American Occupational Therapy Association's (2020) *Occupational Therapy P Framework: Domain and Process, Fourth Edition*. The *Framework* states, "Objective outcomes are measural tangible aspects of improved performance." Screening and assessment tools, along with student case studi support the identification of Tier 2 students who may benefit from these small group interventions. The f ing pages include evidence-based screening and assessment resources that are free or available at a minim These tools assess Tier 2 student issues, including:

- Anxiety
- Bullying
- Depression
- Eating disorders
- Internalizing and externalizing behaviors
- Loneliness
- Mental illness (general)
- Perfectionism
- Self-control
- Self-esteem
- Social-emotional learning
- Subjective well-being
- Substance abuse
- Trauma
- Volition

Reference

American Occupational Therapy Association. (2020). Occupational therapy practice framework: Domain and cess (4th ed.). *American Journal of Occupational Therapy, 74*(Suppl. 2), Article 7412410010. https://doi.org/10 ajot.2020.74S2001

Screening Tools

egory: Anxiety

ening Tool: Preschool Anxiety Scale (PAS)

cription: A 28-item measure using a 5-point Likert scale in which parents report the frequency that an
is true for their child.

Range: Parents of 3- to 5-year-old children

erence: Spence, S. H., Rapee, R., McDonald, C., & Ingram, M. (2001). The structure of anxiety symptoms
ng preschoolers. *Behaviour Research and Therapy, 39*(11), 1293-1316.

---

egory: Anxiety

ening Tool: Revised Children's Anxiety and Depression Scale (RCADS)

cription: A 47-item self-report questionnaire for youth with subscales assessing areas of separation
ety disorder, social phobia, generalized anxiety disorder, panic disorder, obsessive-compulsive disorder,
low mood (major depressive disorder). A parent report form is also available (RCADS-P). A 25-item measure
so available that will screen for broad anxiety symptoms (RCADS-25). RCADS is not recommended for use
youth with moderate or severe learning disabilities. There is an adapted version available for youth with
sm spectrum disorder (ACS-ASD).

Range: 8 to 18 years

erence: Chorpita, B. F., Yim, L. M., Moffitt, C. E., Umemoto L. A., & Francis, S. E. (2000). Assessment of
ptoms of DSM-IV anxiety and depression in children: A Revised Child Anxiety and Depression Scale.
aviour Research and Therapy, 38, 835-855.

---

egory: Anxiety

ening Tool: Screen for Child Anxiety Related Emotional Disorders (SCARED)

scription: This instrument measures anxiety using four domains: panic/somatic, separation anxiety,
eralized anxiety, and school phobia. Child versions and parent versions are available.

Range: 8 to 18 years

ference: Birmaher, B., Brent, D. A., Chiappetta, L., Bridge, J., Monga, S., & Baugher, M. (1999). Psychometric
perties of the Screen for Child Anxiety Related Emotional Disorders (SCARED): A replication study. *Journal
he American Academy of Child and Adolescent Psychiatry, 38*(10), 1230-1236.

Category: Anxiety

Screening Tool: Spence Children's Anxiety Scale (SCAS)

Description: A 44-question scale that assesses the six domains of anxiety, including generalized anxi[...] panic/agoraphobia, social phobia, separation anxiety, obsessive-compulsive disorder, and physical inj[...] fears. Answers are provided on a 4-point Likert scale.

Age Range: 8 to 15 years

Reference: Spence, S. H. (1998). A measure of anxiety symptoms among children. *Behaviour Research [...] Therapy, 36*(5), 545-566.

Category: Anxiety

Screening Tool: Spence Children's Anxiety Scale—Short Version (SCAS-S)

Description: An abbreviated 19-question screen for anxiety.

Age Range: 8 to 15 years

Reference: Ahlen, J., Vigerland, S., & Ghaderi, A. (2018). Development of the Spence Children's Anxiety Sc[...] Short Version (SCAS-S). *Journal of Psychopathology and Behavioral Assessment, 40*(2), 288-304.

Category: Bullying

Screening Tool: Aggression Scale

Description: An 11-item measure assessing frequency of self-reported perpetration of teasing, pushing, [...] threatening others.

Age Range: 10 to 15 years

Reference: Orpinas, P., & Frankowski, R. (2001). The Aggression Scale: A self-report measure of aggress[...] behavior for young adolescents. *Journal of Early Adolescence, 21,* 50-67.

Category: Bullying

Screening Tool: Child Adolescent Bullying Scale (CABS)

Description: A reliable, valid tool for health care providers to screen for bullying exposure.

Age Range: 10 to 17 years

Reference: Strout, T. D., Vessey, J. A., Difazio, R. L., & Ludlow, L. H. (2018). The Child Adolescent Bullying Sca[...] (CABS): Psychometric evaluation of a new measure. *Research in Nursing and Health, 41*(3), 1-13. https://d[...] org/10.1002/nur.21871

egory: Bullying

ening Tool: Peer Interactions in Primary School (PIPS) Questionnaire

cription: The PIPS is the first self-report bullying and victimization measure designed for elementary ol use, which has been determined reliable and valid. The PIPS is a tool that could be used in the design evaluation of school-based bullying and victimization interventions.

Range: Study includes third through sixth graders

rence: Tarshis, T. P., & Huffman, L. C. (2007). Psychometric properties of the Peer Interactions in Primary ol (PIPS) questionnaire. *Journal of Developmental and Behavioral Pediatrics, 28,* 125-132.

---

egory: Depression

ening Tool: Columbia DISC Depression Scale

cription: This screen is available as a teen-report and parent-report, 22 yes/no questions survey. It ers all major mental health diagnoses, and the teen measure also covers suicidal ideation.

Range: 11 years and older

erence: Columbia DISC Development Group of Columbia University. (2008). *Columbia DISC Depression e (ages 11 and over).* Retrieved from http://www.columbia.edu/itc/hs/medical/residency/peds/new_ peds_site/pdfs_new/genpeds_webdocs/Columbia_Depression_Scale_Parent.pdf

---

egory: Depression

eening Tool: Kutcher Adolescent Depression Scale (KADS)

scription: KADS is an 11-item measure that is designed to be sensitive to changes in depression severity time.

Range: 12 to 18 years

erence: Brooks, S. J., Krulewicz, S. P., & Kutcher, S. (2003). The Kutcher Adolescent Depression Scale: essment of its evaluative properties over the course of an 8-week pediatric pharmacotherapy trial. *rnal of Child and Adolescent Psychopharmacology, 13*(3), 337-349.

---

tegory: Depression

eening Tool: Patient Health Questionnaire-9 Item (PHQ-9)

scription: A quick, nine-question screen with high sensitivity and good specificity to detect major pressive disorder in adolescents. This tool can also be used to evaluate the severity of depressive nptoms.

Range: 13 years and older

ference: Richardson, L. P., McCauley, E., Grossman, D. C., McCarty, C. A., Richards, J., Russo, J. E., Rockhill, & Katon, W. (2010). Evaluation of the Patient Health Questionnaire-9 Item for detecting major depression ong adolescents. *Pediatrics, 126*(6), 1117-1123.

Category: Eating Disorders

Screening Tool: Eating Disorder Examination Questionnaire (EDE-Q)

Description: A norm-referenced screen for eating disorders. There is a global score as well as scores restraint subscale, eating concern subscale, weight concern subscale, and shape concern subscale.

Age Range: Original questionnaire can be used for anyone 14 years of age and older; the EDE-A can used for anyone 12 years of age and older

Reference: Mond, J. M., Hay, P. J., Rodgers, B., & Owen, C. (2006). Eating Disorder Examination Questionn. (EDE-Q): Norms for young adult women. *Behaviour Research and Therapy, 44*(1), 53-62.

Category: Internalizing and Externalizing Behaviors

Screening Tool: Locus of Control Scale

Description: A 29-item questionnaire that measures an individual's level of internal-external control.

Age Range: 5 years and older

Reference: Rotter, J. B. (1966). Generalized expectancies for internal versus external control of reinforceme *Psychological Monographs: General and Applied, 80*(1), 1.

Category: Internalizing and Externalizing Behaviors

Screening Tool: Locus of Control Scale for Children

Description: A 40-item yes/no questionnaire measuring the extent to which an individual views control be internal or external.

Age Range: Study includes third through twelfth grades

Reference: Nowicki, S., & Strickland, B. R. (1973). A Locus of Control Scale for Children. *Journal of Consult and Clinical Psychology, 40*(1), 148.

Category: Internalizing and Externalizing Behaviors

Screening Tool: Pediatric Symptom Checklist-17 (PSC-17)

Description: The PSC-17 is frequently used by primary care providers to determine the likelihood th patients have a mental health disorder. The screen can be positive for internalizing behaviors, externalizir behaviors, or attention deficits. Developed by shortening the full PSC that was developed in 1999.

Age Range: 4 to 17 years

Reference: Liu, J., DiStefano, C., Burgess, Y., & Wang, J. (2020). Pediatric Symptom Checklist-17: Testir measurement invariance of a higher-order factor model between boys and girls. *European Journal Psychological Assessment, 36*(1), 77-83. https://doi.org/10.1027/1015-5759/a000495

egory: Internalizing and Externalizing Behaviors

ening Tool: Student Risk Screening Scale—Internalizing and Externalizing (SRSS-IE)

cription: A teacher-report screening tool to evaluate antisocial behaviors of students. These behaviors be internalizing or externalizing.

Range: Versions available for elementary, middle, and high schools

erence: Lane, K. L., Oakes, W. P., Swogger, E. D., Schatschneider, C., Menzies, H. M., & Sanchez, J. (2015). ent Risk Screening Scale for internalizing and externalizing behaviors: Preliminary cut scores to support -informed decision making. *Behavioral Disorders, 40*(3), 159-170.

---

egory: Loneliness

eening Tool: Children's Loneliness Scale

cription: Noted as the gold standard assessment tool of childhood loneliness. A 24-question stionnaire using a 5-point Likert scale.

Range: Originally developed for students in grades 3 through 6; later evidence for use in grades 7 and well as preschool through grade 2

erence: Maes, M., Van den Noortgate, W., Vanhalst, J., Beyers, W., & Goossens, L. (2017). The Children's eliness Scale: Factor structure and construct validity in Belgian children. *Assessment, 24,* 244-251.[a] https:// org/10.1177/1073191115605177. Retrieved from https://successforkidswithhearingloss.com/wp-content/ ads/2011/08/Childrens-Loneliness-and-Social-Dissatisfaction-Scale1.pdf

l created in 1984; this reference is more recent support for the tool.

---

egory: Mental Illness (General)

eening Tool: Columbia Impairment Scale (CIS)—Youth Version

scription: This 13-item instrument is a measure of impairment in a variety of domains, including relations family members, relations with peers, academic functioning, and involvement in personal interests.

Range: 9 to 17 years

ference: Bird, H. R., Shaffer, D., Fisher, P., Gould, M. S., et al. (1993). The Columbia Impairment Scale (CIS): t findings on a measure of global impairment for children and adolescents. *International Journal of thods in Psychiatric Research, 3*(3), 167-176.

---

tegory: Mental Illness (General)

eening Tool: Conners 3 Global Index

scription: A quick, effective screen of general psychopathology. Scores are produced for restlessness- ulsivity, emotional lability, and a total score. There are self-report, parent-report, and teacher-report tions available.

Range: Self-report: 8 to 18 years; parent report: 6 to 18 years

ference: Conners, C. K. (2008). *Connors 3–Parent short form assessment report.* Multi-Health Systems.

Category: Mental Illness (General)

Screening Tool: *Diagnostic and Statistical Manual of Mental Disorders, Fifth Edition* (DSM-5) Cross-Cut[ting] Symptom Measures

Description: This 25-item measure requires the child and parent to report the severity of the ch[ild's] symptoms over the past 2 weeks. This screen serves as a "review of mental systems" (Clarke & Kuhl, 2[014]). There is both a child self-report version and a parent-report version available.

Age Range: Self-report: 11 to 17 years; parent report: 6 to 17 years

Reference: Clarke, D. E., & Kuhl, E. A. (2014). DSM-5 Cross-Cutting Symptom Measures: A step towards [the] future of psychiatric care? *World Psychiatry, 13*(3), 314-316. https://doi.org/10.1002/wps.20154

Category: Mental Illness (General)

Screening Tool: Global Appraisal of Individual Needs–Short Screener (GAIN-SS)

Description: The GAIN-SS is a 16-question survey that evaluates the need for further assessment in [the] areas of mental health, substance abuse, and anger management.

Age Range: Has been used for adolescents as young as 10 years

Reference: Dennis, M. L., Chan, Y. F., & Funk, R. R. (2006). Development and validation of the GAIN Sh[ort] Screener (GSS) for internalizing, externalizing and substance use disorders and crime/violence proble[ms] among adolescents and adults. *American Journal on Addictions, 15,* s80-s91.

Category: Mental Illness (General)

Screening Tool: Kiddie Schedule for Affective Disorders and Schizophrenia—Present and Lifetime Versi[on] (K-SADS-PL)

Description: K-SADS is a very popular measure to screen for most mental illnesses, including ma[jor] depression, mania, hypomania, bipolar disorders, schizoaffective disorders, generalized anxiety disord[er,] obsessive-compulsive disorder, attention-deficit/hyperactivity disorder, oppositional defiant disord[er,] anorexia nervosa, bulimia, Tourette's disorder, substance use disorder, and post-traumatic stress disord[er.] The screening tool consists of completion of the *DSM-5* Cross-Cutting Symptom Measures, an unstructur[ed] interview, and a semistructured screen interview.

Age Range: 6 to 18 years

Reference: Kaufman, J., Birmaher, B., Brent, D., Rao, U., Flynn, C., Moreci, P., Williamson, D., & Ryan, N. (199[7].) Schedule for Affective Disorders and Schizophrenia for school-age children—Present and Lifetime Versi[on] (K-SADS-PL): Initial reliability and validity data. *Journal of the American Academy of Child & Adolescent Psychiat[ry,] 36*(7), 980-988.

egory: Other

ening Tool: Ohio Youth Problems, Functioning, and Satisfaction Scales

cription: This evidence-based set of scales is intended for children who receive mental health services. ns are completed by child, caregiver, and agency worker. Child-report and caregiver-report sections de a Functioning Scale, Hopefulness Scale, Satisfaction Scale, and Problem Severity Scale. The agency cer form substitutes a Restrictiveness of Living Scale for the Hopefulness and Satisfaction Scales.

Range: 5 to 18 years

erence: Ogles, B. M., Melendez, G., Davis, D. C., & Lunnen, K. M. (2000). *The Ohio Youth Problems, tioning, and Satisfaction Scales: Technical manual.* Ohio University.

---

egory: Other

ening Tool: U.S. Department of Education School Climate Survey (EDSCLS)

cription: The School Climate Survey is a comprehensive assessment involving students, staff, and nts to evaluate student engagement, school safety, and the learning environment.

Range: Grades 5 to 12

erence: Wang, Y., Murphy, K., & Kantaparn, C. (2016). Technical and administration user guide for the ED ool Climate Survey (EDSCLS). Retrieved from https://safesupportivelearning.ed.gov/sites/default/files/ CLS%20UserGuide%20042116.pdf

---

egory: Perfectionism

eening Tool: Child-Adolescent Perfectionism Scale (CAPS)

scription: Norm-referenced, 22-question screen that assesses self-oriented perfectionism and socially scribed perfectionism.

Range: 6 to 18 years

erence: Flett, G. L., Hewitt, P. L., Boucher, D. J., Davidson, L. A., & Munro, Y. (1997). Child and Adolescent fectionism Scale (CAPS) [Database record]. *APA PsycTests.* https://doi.org/10.1037/t00787-000

---

tegory: Self-Control

eening Tool: Brief Self-Control Scale (BSCS)

scription: A 13-item scale that evaluates an individual's self-perception of self-control.

Range: Study evaluates high school–aged students

ference: Tangney, J. P., Baumeister, R. F., & Boone, A. L. (2004). High self-control predicts good adjustment, pathology, better grades, and interpersonal success. *Journal of Personality, 72*(2), 271-324.

Category: Self-Esteem

Screening Tool: Rosenberg's Student Self-Esteem Scale

Description: A commonly used 10-item scale to evaluate a student's self-worth. The scale is self-report makes use of a 4-point Likert scale.

Age Range: 12 years and older

Reference: Rosenberg, M. (1965). *Society and the adolescent self-image*. Princeton University Press.

Category: Social-Emotional Learning

Screening Tool: Social Skills Improvement System (SSIS) Rating Scales

Description: The SSIS Rating Scales is designed to assess individuals and small groups to evaluate so skills, problem behaviors, and academic competence. It is hoped that teacher, parent, and student forms provide a comprehensive picture across school, home, and community settings.

Age Range: 3 to 18 years

Reference: Gresham, F. M., & Elliott, S. N. (2008). *Social Skills Improvement System Rating Scales manual.* N Pearson.

Category: Social-Emotional Learning

Screening Tool: Strengths and Difficulties Questionnaire (SDQ)

Description: A 25-question screen to evaluate strengths and weakness in the areas of emotional sympton conduct problems, hyperactivity, inattention, peer relationship problems, and prosocial behaviors. T screen is available in many languages, including Spanish and French. Administration involves parent teacher (self-report version available for children ages 11 to 16 years).

Age Range: Versions available that are appropriate for those 3 to 16 years of age. Versions listed at http: www.sdqinfo.org/py/sdqinfo/b3.py?language=Englishqz (USA).

Reference: Goodman, R. (1997). The Strengths and Difficulties Questionnaire: A research note. *Journal Child Psychology and Psychiatry, 38*(5), 581-586.

Category: Subjective Well-Being

Screening Tool: Brief Multidimensional Students' Life Satisfaction Scale (BMSLSS)

Description: The BMSLSS is a reliable, five-item tool to screen for life satisfaction of students.

Age Range: 8 to 18 years

Reference: Seligson, J. L., Huebner, E. S., & Valois, R. F. (2003). Preliminary validation of the Br Multidimensional Students' Life Satisfaction Scale (BMSLSS). *Social Indicators Research, 61*(2), 121-145.

gory: Subjective Well-Being

ening Tool: EPOCH Measure of Adolescent Well-Being

cription: The EPOCH Measure of Adolescent Well-Being evaluates five positive psychological qualities: gement, perseverance, optimism, connectedness, and happiness. The adolescent rates the frequency which 20 statements are true on a scale of 1 to 5.

Range: 10 to 18 years

rence: Kern, M. L., Benson, L., Steinberg, E. A., & Steinberg, L. (2016). The EPOCH Measure of Adolescent -Being. *Psychological Assessment, 28*(5), 586.

---

egory: Subjective Well-Being

ening Tool: Multidimensional Students' Life Satisfaction Scale (MSLSS)

cription: The MSLSS is a 40-item scale that assesses six different dimensions of a student's life faction using a 6-point Likert scale.

Range: 8 to 18 years

erence: Huebner, E. S. (1994). Preliminary development and validation of a multidimensional life faction scale for children. *Psychological Assessment, 6*(2), 149.

---

egory: Substance Abuse

ening Tool: CRAFFT Screening Tool for Adolescent Substance Use

cription: A short assessment tool designed to screen for substance-related risks and problems in lescents.

Range: 12 to 21 years

erence: Knight, J. R., Shrier, L. A., Bravender, T. D., Farrell, M., Vander Bilt, J., & Shaffer, H. J. (1999). A new brief en for adolescent substance abuse. *Archives of Pediatrics & Adolescent Medicine, 153*(6), 591-596.

---

tegory: Trauma

ening Tool: Pediatric Adverse Childhood Events (ACEs) and Related Life Event Screener (PEARLS)

cription: A 17-item instrument with high face validity and acceptability for use within primary care tings to screen for pediatric ACEs.

Range: The PEARLS child tool is for ages 0 to 11 years and is completed by a parent/caregiver. The RLS adolescent tool is for ages 12 to 19 years and is completed by a parent/caregiver and by the lescent.

ference: Koita, K., Long, D., Hessler, D., Benson, M., Daley, K., Bucci, M., Thakur, N., & Harris, N. B. (2018). velopment and implementation of a pediatric adverse childhood experiences (ACEs) and other erminants of health questionnaire in the pediatric medical home: A pilot study. *PLoS One, 13*(12), 208088. https://doi.org/10.1371/journal.pone.0208088

Assessment Tools

Assessment Tool: Child Occupational Self Assessment (COSA)

Authors: Kramer, ten Velden, Kafkes, Basu, Federico, and Kielhofner

Format: Rating form with pictures, rating form without pictures, or card sort

Purpose: To determine a child's perception of their occupational competence and its importance rela
to typically performed occupations.

Population: 7 to 17 years

Time Required: 25 minutes

Description: The COSA is a self-report assessment that evaluates a child's perception of their occupatic
competence and the relative importance of typically performed occupations. Occupations at school, in
home, and in the community are assessed. The version 2.2 manual includes three administration options
support the client in completing the assessment successfully. The options include a card sort, a self-rat
form with symbols, and a self-rating form without symbols.

Source: MOHO Clearinghouse—University of Illinois at Chicago (https://moho-irm.uic.edu/default.aspx)

Cost: $40

Reference: Keller, J., Kafkes, A., Basu, S., Federico, J., & Kielhofner, G. (2006). *A user's manual for the Cl
Occupational Self Assessment (COSA) (v. 2.1).* Model of Human Occupation Clearinghouse. Department
Occupational Therapy, College of Applied Health Sciences, University of Illinois at Chicago.

Assessment Tool: Occupational Therapy Psychosocial Assessment of Learning (OT PAL)

Authors: Townsend, University of Illinois at Chicago

Format: Observation and interview

Purpose: To determine best fit between a child and the school environment.

Population: 6 to 12 years

Time Required: Variable

Description: The OT PAL is completed through observation and interviews to evaluate a student's volitic
habituation, and environmental fit within the classroom setting.

Source: MOHO Clearinghouse—University of Illinois at Chicago (https://moho-irm.uic.edu/default.aspx)

Cost: $40

Reference: Townsend, S., Carey, P., Hollins, N., Helfrich, C., Blondis, M., Hoffman, A., Collins, L., Knudson,
& Blackwell, A. (2001). *A user's manual for Occupational Therapy Psychosocial Assessment of Learning (OT PA
Version 2.0.* Model of Human Occupation Clearinghouse, Department of Occupational Therapy, College
Applied Health Sciences, University of Illinois at Chicago.

essment Tool: Pediatric Volitional Questionnaire (PVQ)

hors: Basu, Kafkes, Schatz, Kiraly, and Kielhofner

mat: Observational assessment

pose: Assess volitional development of a child within their environment.

ulation: 2 to 7 years

e Required: 30 minutes

cription: The PVQ is an observational assessment that can be used to evaluate a child's motivation in their environment. A child's volitional development is assessed in the stages of exploration, petency, and achievement.

rce: MOHO Clearinghouse—University of Illinois at Chicago (https://moho-irm.uic.edu/default.aspx)

t: $40

erence: Basu, S., Kafkes, A., Schatz, R., Kiraly, A., & Kielhofner, G. (2008). *A user's manual for the Pediatric ional Questionnaire (Version 2.1)*. Model of Human Occupation Clearinghouse, Department of Occupational apy, College of Applied Health Sciences, University of Illinois at Chicago.

---

essment Tool: School Setting Interview (SSI)

hors: Hemmingsson, Egilson, Hoffman, and Kielhofner

mat: Semistructured interview

pose: To determine potential mismatch between a student and the educational environment and mote involvement in appropriate school activities.

ulation: 6 years and older

e Required: 40 minutes

scription: The SSI is designed to identify the misfits between a student and their environment. environments in which the child assumes a student role are considered, including the classroom, ground, and gymnasium, as well as hallways and field trips. The purpose of this assessment is to ermine if a student's current accommodations are satisfactory or if additional accommodations and/or stive technology should be implemented to maximize occupational performance.

irce: MOHO Clearinghouse—University of Illinois at Chicago (https://moho-irm.uic.edu/default.aspx)

st: $40

erence: Hemmingsson, H., Egilson, S., Hoffman, O., & Kielhofner, G. (2005). *A user's manual for the School ting Interview (SSI) (v.3.0)*. Model of Human Occupation Clearinghouse, Department of Occupational erapy, College of Applied Health Sciences, University of Illinois at Chicago.

Assessment Tool: Short Child Occupational Profile (SCOPE)

Authors: Bowyer, Kramer, Ploszaj, Ross, Schwartz, Kielhofner, and Kramer

Format: Occupation-based performance measure

Purpose: To describe occupational participation in terms of strengths and challenges; screener occupational therapy services.

Population: Birth to 21 years

Time Required: 15 to 20 minutes

Description: The SCOPE is designed to be a systematic evaluation of most concepts in the MOHO mo It can be completed through observation of the child, interviews of parents or teachers, chart review, a other assessments. The child's strengths and challenges are assessed in the areas of volition, habituati and performance skills. The SCOPE also evaluates the extent to which the environment facilitates restricts occupational participation. Twenty-five items are organized into six sections: volition, habituati communication and interaction, process skills, motor skills, and impact of environment.

Source: MOHO Clearinghouse—University of Illinois at Chicago (https://moho-irm.uic.edu/default.aspx)

Cost: $40

Reference: Bowyer, P. L., Kramer, J., Ploszaj, A., Ross, M., Schwartz, O., Kielhofner, G., & Kramer, K. (2005). *A us manual for the Short Child Occupational Profile (SCOPE) (v.2.2)*. Model of Human Occupation Clearinghou Department of Occupational Therapy, College of Applied Health Sciences, University of Illinois at Chicag

Section 3

Occupational Therapy Groups

Group #1

Pam Stephenson, OTD, OTR/L, BCP, FAOTA

GROUP TITLE	Fortunately Teller: What Can I Say or Do?
ACTIVITY	Paper craft/origami
PURPOSE	The purpose of this group activity is to help students make better choices for managing anger and frustration at school. The group reinforces that, **fortunately we can make different choices** and practice responding and participating in new ways at school. Each group member makes a paper fortune teller to identify different things they can **fortunately say or do** to manage anger at school pre-emptively and/ or when frustrating events occur. The group uses a craft occupation to invite students to explore new self-management strategies and how the fortune teller can be used as a tool to begin developing new habits that replace externalizing behaviors with acceptable and alternative school behaviors they can **fortunately say or do**. Consider this small group intervention when the problem-solving team has student concerns about any of the following occupational issues: • Feeling overwhelmed by anger and acting out • Being aggressive with others • Damaging school property • Breaking classroom rules • Having difficulty coping with anger • Feeling that consequences at school are outside of one's personal control

SESSION GOALS	1. Make a fortune teller craft. 2. Identify different things that can be **fortunately said or done**. 3. Strategize how the fortune teller could be used in different school situations during the day. 4. Role play and practice using the fortune teller in hypothetical school situations
OCCUPATION AS MEANS AND ENDS	This group uses a craft to support making more appropriate activity and behavior choices and developing habits that lead to effective behavior change(s) at school.
DIRECTIONS	This activity is envisioned to be part of a small group check-in/check-out program t͟ support learners to develop habits around making better behavioral choices at sch͟ To begin the group, the members should brainstorm a list of activities they can do at school when they feel angry or before participating in a situation that has been historically frustrating. The occupational therapy practitioner can help to generate t͟ list of things that students can "**fortunately say or do** without breaking classroom or school rules." Next, each group member should follow the folding instructions to make a paper fortune teller. Many different online resources provide step-by-step folding instructions (e.g., www.easypeasyandfun.com/how-to-make-a-fortune-teller/). Each member can customize their craft according to the strategies that they feel will work best and based on personal activity preferences. The occupational therapy practitioner also reinforces that the ultimate goal is to use the fortune teller throughout the day to either respond to situations that make them feel angry or overwhelmed. Students have a chance to practice in different role play situations. Upon check-out, students report on how well they managed their frustration and used the fortune teller during that school day.
MATERIALS	• Blank sheets of paper (one for each student; preprinted fortune teller sheets are available for purchase or could be preprinted) • Colored pens, crayons • Scissors
MESSY FACTOR	Low
PINTEREST TERMS	Free paper fortune teller templates, DIY fortune teller game, cootie catcher origami
GRADE LEVEL	Elementary school

essing the Group: Tip Sheet

troduction and Warm-Up Ideas

ainstorm situations at school that are most frustrating (incorporate into role play scenarios later)
d and watch a video on making a paper fortune teller to prepare them for the activity
quick fill-in-the-blank to: "If I get frustrated while trying to do this activity, **fortunately I can say or do**
_____."
ake a list of classroom and school rules that group members may be struggling with

ays to Grade or Modify the Activity

ve premade or prefolded fortune tellers
nt out the step-by-step directions or show a video
ve a predetermined list of adaptive behaviors and choices for handling anger and frustration at school that
incide with school expectations

uestions You May Want to Ask

ow does managing your frustration and anger help you to do the things you need to do at school?
ow might you use this fortune teller to help you complete your tasks and accomplish your goals at school?
hat kinds of things may people notice about you when you are following school rules consistently? How do
u think they will describe you as a student?
ow will your behavior at school change if you try hard to use this tool throughout the day? How will that
lp you be a better friend? Student? Member of the class?
hich activities could you do at school to help you feel more calm and less frustrated or angry?
ow does this fortune teller help you develop the habit of thinking before you act?
ow may the fortune teller help you feel more confident that you can follow the school/classroom rules?
hich people at school can help you pick things that you can **fortunately say or do**?
is activity helped you think of things you can **fortunately say or do** before you act in anger or frustration.
ow well did you do? What skills will you use the next time you feel angry or frustrated at school?

acilitation Strategies

ovide students with practice during role play scenarios based on situations that typically make them feel
ustrated or angry
elp them understand the importance of using the fortune teller before they feel angry or frustrated

Facilitator's Notes

- What students noted makes them frustrated or angry at school

- Ideas of how to use it pre-emptively or prior to participation in a school task that is normally frustrati

- How the toy supports self-management

- Habits related to thinking before you act/respond

Group #2

Anne Kiraly-Alvarez, OTD, OTR/L, SCSS
and Nashauna (Neki) Richardson, EdD, MS, OTR/L

GROUP TITLE	Jumping to the BETTER Conclusions: Checkers
ACTIVITY	Board game
	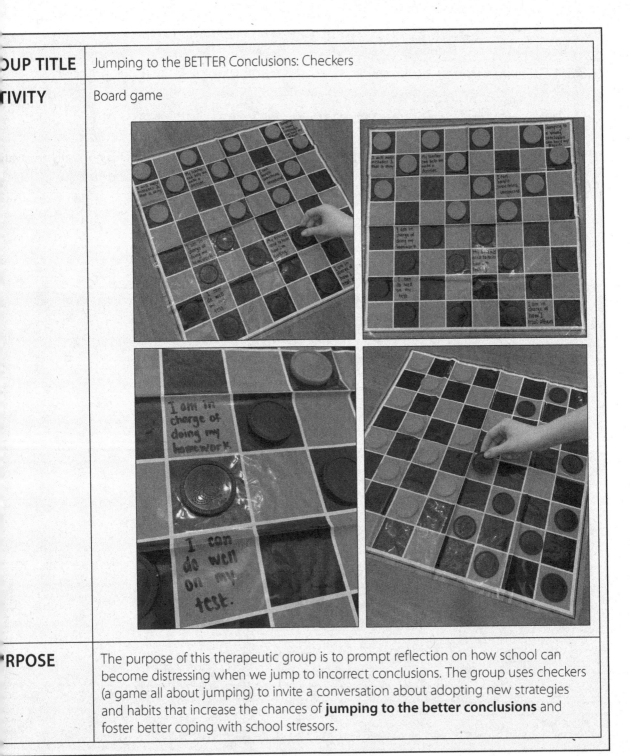
PURPOSE	The purpose of this therapeutic group is to prompt reflection on how school can become distressing when we jump to incorrect conclusions. The group uses checkers (a game all about jumping) to invite a conversation about adopting new strategies and habits that increase the chances of **jumping to the better conclusions** and foster better coping with school stressors.

	Consider this small group intervention when the problem-solving team has studen concerns about any of the following occupational issues: • Blames others for their own mistakes on school tasks • Expects negative or poor academic outcomes • Has decreased coping when school situations change or shift • Does not effectively accept responsibilities associated with being a student, pe or friend (school roles) • Struggles with peer relationships because they expect others to read their min
SESSION GOALS	1. Play different variations of checkers. 2. Explore how the rules for jumping and capturing are different in each variation. 3. Identify strategies that help with **jumping to the better conclusions**.
OCCUPATION AS MEANS AND ENDS	This group involves playing checkers (learning new ways to jump and capture) to invite students to explore new strategies and habits that will help them jump to the right conclusions.
DIRECTIONS	**Phase 1:** Students are asked to play checkers according to the traditional rules of the game. Checkers was chosen because the process for jumping pieces follows a predictable order and direction. **Phase 2:** Students play a different variation of checkers that incorporates different rules for making jumps and capturing. The international variation of checkers allows for checker pieces to move forward and backward and jump in either direction. The flying kings variation allows kings to move any number of open spaces along a diagonal. Italian checkers does not permit checker pieces to jump kings. Polish checkers allows a player to continue making subsequent jumps after a checker becomes a king if they are available. Participants process the here and now of having played variations of checkers and adapting to a new set of rules for jumping and capturing pieces. Specifically, they explore how they might apply this experience to developing a new set of rules to help them more likely **jump to a better conclusion**, rather than jumping to a wron conclusion.
MATERIALS	• Checkers game • Rule changer cards (included)
MESSY FACTOR	Low
PINTEREST TERMS	DIY LEGO checkerboard, rock checkers crafts, checkers
GRADE LEVEL	Middle school (but could be adapted for elementary and high schools)

essing the Group: Tip Sheet

troduction and Warm-Up Ideas

gressively reveal frames of photos and images to demonstrate how we may **jump to incorrect conclu-
ns** when we do not have the full picture

ntify times at school **when jumping to the wrong conclusion** had a personal or significant impact

ke a simple checkerboard out of construction paper that can be used to play the game

ve the group brainstorm the rules for traditional checkers on the board or poster

ays to Grade or Modify the Activity

minate option of playing checkers by traditional rules and jump into new variations

int out rules of the game to reinforce how the rules can help guide actions

uestions You May Want to Ask

w will checking assumptions and facts help you **jump to better conclusions?**

hat skills were you using when you played the game with new rules? How will those skills help you to **jump
better conclusions?**

w do you imagine your relationships with friends, peers, and teachers will change if your process for
mping to better conclusions** improves?

ho might be able to help you check your facts and assumptions at school so that you are more likely going
jump to a better conclusion? What kinds of questions might you ask them?

w will you practice these problem-solving skills so that you can do them automatically when you have a
uation at school?

acilitation Strategies

ormalize that everyone usually does not have all the information they need for decisions

elp them to understand how the **jumping to the wrong conclusions** has created issues for them at school

xplore ways to respond when we may have **jumped to the wrong conclusion** and need to change our minds
d **jump to a better (new) conclusion**

Facilitator's Notes

- Ideas and strategies for generating workable solutions and drawing conclusions

- How changing the rules of the checkers game invited them to be open to new ways for themselves

- How poor problem solving has created school issues for the group members

Group #3

*Susan Friguglietti, DHA, MA, OTR/L
and Mark Bumgarner, MS*

GROUP TITLE	Changing Your Tune With a Little **Care**-a-oke
ACTIVITY	Singing/musical game
PURPOSE	This group invites participants to listen to music, experiment with creative songwriting, and have a **care**-a-oke sing off to get **in tune** with what they most care about. Students describe how those values and interests fit into their life story and how they possibly feel stuck at school. Additionally, the group addresses ambivalence and supports self-efficacy so students can begin to see a path for how they can **change their tune** about school. Group members also collectively explore how they could make different activity and occupational choices at school to make the experience seem more meaningful and help them **change their tune** about school. This Tier 2 group might be best for students with the following occupational issues: • Limited motivation to complete school work on time and earn higher grades • Lack of persistence to complete school tasks because they do not seem meaningful • Limited interest in school and student role, especially if they are uncertain about how it fits into future goals, which may increase risk for dropping out • Do not expect good or meaningful things to happen at school
SESSION GOALS	1. Play a few rounds of **care**-a-oke. 2. Identify issues that seem to limit motivation to go to school or complete school tasks. 3. Values clarification and exploration (identify what the group member cares about).
OCCUPATION AS MEANS AND ENDS	This group uses singing as a means to encourage making activity choices based on personal values/interests so that going to school becomes more personally meaningful.

DIRECTIONS	**Phase 1:** Participants are instructed to identify a song about something they care about deeply. Under the facilitator's supervision, each student locates a song lyric video and plays the lyrics that matter the most for the larger group. Time constrain may only provide an opportunity for each group member to play short snippets.
	Phase 2: Participants are asked to literally change their tune by superimposing the lyrics of their chosen song with the melody of a popular tune they roll on the cube (i.e., sing "Shake It Off" to the tune of "Mary Had a Little Lamb"). The group will likely find this task to be quite difficult, which can be normalized later when discussing the challenges of making meaningful changes in our lives. After several minutes of songwriting, the group votes on who **changed their tune** the best in a lively versic of **care**-a-oke. It is possible that some tunes may even sound pretty good!
MATERIALS	• Technology and internet access • Song cube (example provided) • Song lyrics (approved by facilitator)
MESSY FACTOR	Low
PINTEREST TERMS	Paper dice template, behavior change plan, motivational interviewing
GRADE LEVEL	Middle and high schools

Example Song Cube Template

To use the song cube, cut out the following, fold across the lines, and tape to form a die.

	Jingle Bells	
Happy Birthday Song	Take Me Out To The Ballgame	Star Spangled Banner
	Auld Lang Syne	
	Mary Had A Little Lamb	

essing the Group: Tip Sheet

troduction and Warm-Up Ideas

are song choices and the lyrics or themes that are personally most meaningful

ve the group discuss the difference between these two questions: "What's the matter with you?" and "What tters to you?"

ays to Grade or Modify the Activity

nsider allowing students to print out the lyrics to their songs

nsider singing as a group instead of individually

ve the students only rewrite the harmony for the main refrain of the song or the particular lyrics that were entified as having personal meaning

uestions You May Want to Ask

hat strategies helped the most for **changing your tune**? How might those strategies support you in ap-aching school behavior differently?

what extent can you relate your future goals to what you are being asked to do at school right now?

hat might the school experience be like for you if it included more opportunities to participate and engage activities you personally value?

w does acting in ways that are consistent with your values support your goals and the things you men-ned matter to you?

w confident are you that you can make the changes necessary to get more enjoyment from your school periences?

hat is the next step for you in terms of **changing your tune** about school?

acilitation Strategies

ake sure to be mindful and approve all lyrics

sten for any change talk in their statements; refer to the DARN CAT acronym (desire, ability, reason, need, mmitment, activation, taking steps) in motivational interviewing

ormalize the parts of change that can be difficult—there is ambivalence and changing motivation; the urse is often nonlinear

Facilitator's Notes

- Group comments that supported change talk

- How occupation encouraged meaningful participation

- Ways you linked the literal change work in the activity with the figurative change work necessary fo proved occupational competence and participation

Group #4

Meaghan Smeraglia, MOT, OTR/L, CCA

GROUP TITLE	Flow Before You Throw
ACTIVITY	Darts
PURPOSE	This small group explores the relationship between recent concerns about school and personal difficulties with feeling overwhelmed and acting impulsively. Participants use darts (or Velcro ball toss) to build emotional awareness and practice self-regulation techniques that help them get in the **flow before they throw** (i.e., think before they act). Additionally, the group intervention addresses how we can build our self-efficacy by being intentional in how we position ourselves to successfully hit our targets. This Tier 2 group may be particularly helpful for students who may: • Have positive screens for being overwhelmed at school • Express a low sense of self-efficacy • Have difficulty following school or classroom expectations • Act impulsively or defiantly with teachers • Have decreased coping and adapting to changes at school • Have restricted activity choices based on fear of failure

SESSION GOALS	1. Play darts or target toss mindfully.
	2. Find pleasure in participating in a school activity.
	3. Identify strategies to relax and concentrate before they throw so they increase chances of hitting their target.
OCCUPATION AS MEANS AND ENDS	Use darts to practice self-regulation and examine how they can use this experience develop a new process that increases the likelihood of hitting their targets and get the results that matter most to them at school.
DIRECTIONS	During this game, students take turns throwing at a dart board. Each turn, the playe gets two rounds with three tosses in each round. During the first round, the player throws quickly and spontaneously three times. Before their second round, the playe pulls a card from the "flow" deck. The card they pull could be determined by where their dart lands on a color-coded board, or that card could be pulled at random. Th flow deck includes the following categories:
	• **F**: Feel (building emotional and body awareness)
	• **L**: Learn (practicing self-regulation skills)
	• **O**: Outcome (identifying goals)
	• **W**: Words (using supportive language)
	The player practices the flow activity, and then throws their last round of three tosses. This may be followed by a brief discussion to process whether the student or class noticed a difference in their ability to reach the target after the flow round. This discussion can broaden, touching on areas outside of the darts game where th student could apply the concepts of self-regulation to support goal achievement within the student role.
MATERIALS	• Dart game or Velcro ball toss game
	• Flow cards (included)
	• Optional: Tape to mark standing line, notecards, writing utensils
MESSY FACTOR	Low
PINTEREST TERMS	Throw/toss games, mindfulness techniques, grounding activities, self-regulation strategies, coping skills, self-talk, impulse control, self-efficacy
GRADE LEVEL	Middle school (but could be adapted for elementary and high schools)

le Feel Cards

el Cards tional awareness: What emotion am I feeling? Where do I feel it? What do I want to feel?)		
emotion do you feel now? Name it! Thank it. go. ember a time you felt **idence**. Focus on the g of **confidence**. Now, v with **confidence**.	What emotion do you feel right now? Name it! Thank it. Let it go. Remember a time you felt **joy**. Focus on the feeling of **joy**. Now, throw with **joy**.	How would you define a personal warning sign? What are three warning signs you have when you feel **anxious**? Ask for help if you need it to come up with ideas!
t emotion do you feel now? Name it! Thank it. go. ember a time you felt **ud** of yourself. Focus on eeling of **pride**. Now, v with **pride**.	What emotion do you feel right now? Name it! Thank it. Let it go. Remember a time you felt **relaxed**. Focus on the feeling of being **relaxed**. Now, throw **relaxed**.	When you are about to lose control, what warning signs do you notice about your: **Body:** Do you have a fast heartbeat, get sweaty, or begin to shake? **Mind:** Do you think negative thoughts, curse, or feel bad about yourself?
t emotion do you feel now? Name it! Thank it. t go. ember a time you felt **eful**. Focus on the ng of **hope**. Now, throw **hope**.	What emotion do you feel right now? Name it! Thank it. Let it go. Remember a time you felt **excited**. Focus on the feeling of **excitement**. Now, throw with **excitement**.	Give an example of when you acted impulsively/ without thinking. How do you think **other** people feel when you act this way?

Sample Learn Cards

L: Learn Cards (Self-regulation strategies: What can I do to regulate, relax, and focus?)		
Visualize Close your eyes or look at the board. Like a movie, imagine the dart or ball landing on the target three times.	**Pose** Strike a yoga pose of your choice. Hold for three breaths. Take audience suggestions if needed!	**Heat** Put your hands together. Slide them up and down quickly, creating heat with your hands. Place your wa[rm] hands on your face or bo[dy] feeling the temperature change.
Breathe Breathe in through your nose for two counts and breath out through your mouth making a "HAAAAA" sound for as long as you can comfortably. Do three times. Bonus if you make it loud! Double bonus if you laugh!	**Stretch** Do a body stretch of your choice. Hold for three breaths.	**Temples** Look at the bullseye with laser-focused eyes or close your eyes and imagine it. Bring both your hands up next to your face. Rub or tap your fingers over your temples (next to your eye[s]). Do for three breaths.
Squeeze Relax your body and inhale. Now squeeze every muscle in your body at once, even your toes! Hold your breath for three counts. Relax your body and exhale. Repeat three times.	**Shake** Give yourself permission to be silly and embrace being "weird" as a badge of honor. Shake and wiggle out your body. Shake out your feet, legs, hips, arms, hands, shoulders, and head. You can hop and jump too. Get the whole class up and moving!	**Press** Cross your arms across you[r] chest like a mummy. Press your middle and pointer fingers down under your collarbone and hold for th[ree] breaths.

ble Outcome Cards

utcome Cards
tifying goals: What is my goal?)

ribe where you want the to land on the board.	What small change can you make in the way you toss this next throw to improve your chances of hitting the target?	Ask the audience for advice on how you can improve your throw. Try it out!
e a time when you eved something you r thought you could.	Share a time when you earned a really great grade on a challenging assignment.	Share about one person who helps you achieve your school goals.
cribe what you think the strategy is for getting a eye.	Describe one way you can take care of yourself every day to succeed as a student.	How can you cope if you do not accomplish your goals?

Sample Word Cards

W: Word Cards		
(Supportive self-talk: What helpful and motivating words can I say to myself?)		
Say this phrase confidently three times in your head or aloud: "I can do hard things!"	Say this phrase kindly three times in your head or aloud: "I believe in myself!"	Say this phrase proudly th[ree] times in your head or alou[d] "I am learning!"
Share three compliments you have received from others this past year.	What is your go-to motivational quote? Say it in your head or aloud three times.	What is an unkind though[t] you have about yourself a[ ]lot? What is a kinder thing you can say to yourself? Phone a friend for help if needed!
List three things you are proud of yourself for doing this week.	What is your go-to motivational song lyric? Say it in your head or aloud three times.	What is an unkind stateme[nt] someone has said about you that you have never forgotten? What is a kinder phrase or thought you can say to yourself instead?

essing the Group: Tip Sheet

troduction and Warm-Up Ideas

llaborate with students to generate game rules (do not step over the fault line, do not distract peers during ir turn, and be open to trying new things)

eate ice breaker questions, where the students share their small and big academic goals

plore with the students' situations where they act without thinking in school

ite the flow categories on the board and have the students brainstorm examples

ve students pick one of the flow categories and write an example on a notecard to add to the deck before ying

ays to Grade or Modify the Activity

e a Velcro ball toss game or magnetic darts instead of a traditional dart board

move the first round of throws altogether, having the students start their turns by reading the flow cards d then tossing

crease or decrease the number of throws and standing distance from the board

ve the students lead their classmates in whichever flow card they selected to increase social participation d comfortability being vulnerable

grade by encouraging students to make up their own flow ideas and create DIY flow cards the students n take with them after the group

rm teams, keep score, and award prizes for increased opportunities to practice expected social skills

ve the students ask their peers follow-up questions during the discussion

lapt the language and activities on the flow cards to suit students' needs; for example, edit the Learn cards have catchy names (e.g., "Dragon Breath" for breathing technique)

uestions You May Want to Ask

ere you able to find enjoyment in the game, even if you did not hit your target? Where in your life can you actice enjoying the process more, without being overly tied to getting a "bullseye"?

hat coping strategies can you use to support yourself if you do not achieve your target?

hat school activities and situations make you have big feelings and lead you to react without thinking?

hich flow skills or coping strategies can you use to help you relax and focus before taking action?

id you notice a difference between throwing before and after practicing a flow skill? How might you be able use this skill to hit your targets at school?

hat targets do you want to reach in school? Which flow skills can help you reach those targets?

here in your everyday routine could you start using flow skills to help you meet your goals? How can you ake this a habit or daily ritual?

acilitation Strategies

ocus on how building awareness of one's feelings, thoughts, and warning signs give students the power to be control and choose their actions to achieve their goals

einforce using coping skills, positive self-talk, and having self-compassion when not achieving the desired esults

ocus on both the importance of taking steps toward achieving their goals, while simultaneously having flex-ility regarding the outcome

imply find enjoyment in the process of doing an occupation

Normalize that everyone misses the target at times

Facilitator's Notes

- How self-awareness and regulation are essential for optimal occupational participation and goal achiev

- How occupation encouraged participation and supported self-efficacy

- How you processed what happened in the group with what might happen in other school-based situat

- The strategies that helped accuracy

Group #5

Wanda Mahoney, PhD, OTR/L, FAOTA
and Brad E. Egan, OTD, PhD, CADC, OTR/L

GROUP TITLE	Daily Positivity: **Accordion** to Me
ACTIVITY	Bookbinding

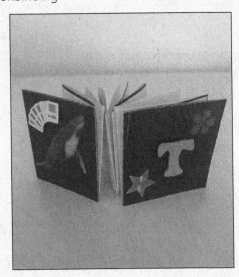 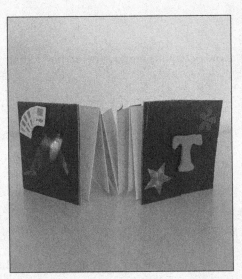

PURPOSE	"What makes life awesome?" is a question that prompts reflection. This can sometimes be a difficult question to answer, especially for students who do not feel effective and do not anticipate success with school tasks or school relationships. The purpose of this group is to make a small, portable, **accordion-style** book to prompt students to identify aspects of their school day and performance that, **accordion to them**, are positive.

Blank pages in the book provide daily opportunities to build habits around appraising their skills and values, practice gratitude, build their confidence to adapt and cope to stressful or changing situations at school, affirm oneself, and choose activities that they want to be able to participate in more or perform better. Students are expected to carry the book with them around school and fill out the prompts as they occur during the day.

The group may be helpful for students who:

- Avoid challenges for fear of making a mistake or not being perfect

- Have trouble appraising their abilities

- Limit themselves to activity choices that are too easy relative to their skills

- Have difficulty using their strengths and skills to cope adaptively to difficult situations at school

	• Present with limited self-efficacy
	• Struggle to express pride
	• Present with an external locus of control and need encouragement to make choices based on what is important **accordion to them**
SESSION GOALS	1. Complete and bind a small accordion book. 2. Answer the prompts so each student has a worked example. 3. Discuss the value of repetition for creating new habits. 4. Discuss how to use the book during the school day.
OCCUPATION AS MEANS AND ENDS	This bookbinding group offers students an opportunity to make a mini (portable) accordion book. Students then use the book over the next few weeks to develop n habits at school.
DIRECTIONS	Students use the templates provided to make the front and back covers of the mini book and the accordion pages. Fold along all the columns and rows and cut along the darkened lines. Use a glue stick or a quick-drying glue to adhere the pages to the front and back covers. Consider encouraging the students to decorate the covers with symbols, words, quotes, or messages that reflect a personal goal or something positive. Once the covers are adhered, there should be a total of 30 blan squares or pages if both sides are counted. Each square represents a daily challenge perhaps there are enough to encourage new self-affirming behaviors to become more automatic. Once a day, students should reflect on their day and complete the following prompts on one page: 1) a skill I used today, 2) an activity that was personally meaningful today, 3) something I am grateful for today, and 4) a statemer of self-affirmation. **Example Page** *Creativity* *Eating lunch with Lucy* *Sunshine* *I am brave* *Try out for play* The facilitator can design different prompts or page styles. Be creative!

TERIALS	• Cardboard pieces • Paper • Glue stick or tape • Markers, paint, and art supplies to decorate the book covers • Ribbon to bind the book/rubber band
SSY :TOR	Low
TEREST RMS	Mini accordion books, origami, origami mini book, rubber band book binding, one-word journal prompts, self-affirmation lists
ADE 'EL	High school (prompts could be adapted for elementary and middle schools)

Trace this square on cardboard or thicker stock material for the front and back covers.

Cut along the darkened lines after folding the paper along all the rows and all the columns.

...essing the Group: Tip Sheet

...troduction and Warm-Up Ideas

...view examples of self-affirmations and different skills that support positive mental well-being

...nd an inspirational quote or two and write them on the book covers

...are and explain the personal significance of each quote chosen

...ays to Grade or Modify the Activity

...ter the number of rows and columns to either increase or decrease the number of days students address ...ese prompts

...ve students fill out a few pages a day by reflecting at different times (e.g., once in the morning, at midday, ...d before bed)

...e different prompts

...uestions You May Want to Ask

...hat kinds of activities usually put you in a positive and/or hopeful mood at school?

...hat activities and skills have you practiced in the past that led to you becoming more skilled? How can that ...me approach apply to practicing wellness?

...hat activities do you think you will be successful doing at school next year?

...ow do you use your skills in more than one activity at school? Which skills do you seem to be using the ...ost during the school day?

...hat are some strategies you will use to remember to write in your book each day for the next month?

...ow do you imagine that you will take care of your book?

...acilitation Strategies

...ncourage students to review their posts on a regular basis

...onsider having a poster or handout of a variety of different self-affirmations

...einforce the portability of the mini reflection book so they can use it when they feel they need a moment of ...ncouragement during the school day or at home

...iscuss strategies that make habits stick and explore when they have had previous successes changing or ...dopting a new habit

Facilitator's Notes

- Statements that suggest expectations of success

- Ways that occupations were discussed to encourage wellness and develop habits

- Considerations for how the book can serve as a daily tool when a student may need to feel encouraged

Group #6

Toymika LeFlore, MEd, OTR/L

GROUP TITLE	Keeping Life in the Balance: Centering and Grounding
ACTIVITY	Craft
PURPOSE	Students complete a centerpiece (craft) that needs to be **centered and grounded**. The techniques that were used to ground the Mylar helium balloons into the centerpiece and those that were used to center the piece to keep it from toppling over are explored as possible ways to build **centering and grounding** practices into one's daily routine at school.

Occupation-focused problem solving can help students to recognize different occupations that may help with being more centered and/or grounded. Moreover, strategies can be discussed for incorporating these occupations into their daily routine so they adapt better to the demands and expectations of student role.

This Tier 2 group may be helpful for students whose screening results indicate:

- Feeling **imbalanced** or without a helpful routine
- Mental fatigue owing to recurring and overwhelming emotions (dread, anger, worry) at school
- Increased stress during the school day or when engaging in school-related activities
- Not meeting student role obligations in a socially and personally acceptable manner
- Do not feel supported at school
- Unable to concentrate negatively impacts academic performance

SESSION GOALS	1. Create a plan for making a centerpiece that addresses how the design keeps the helium balloons from flying away (**grounding**) and keeps the structure from leaning or toppling over (**centering**).
	2. Encourage students to identify parallels between the strategies they used to **center and ground** the centerpiece and the strategies that could be used to build a routine at school incorporating activities that are personally **centering and grounding**.
OCCUPATION AS MEANS AND ENDS	Students complete a craft and use the here-and-now experience to make a plan for new routine at school.
DIRECTIONS	Students are given at least one filled Mylar helium balloon, several different-sized traditional balloons, curling ribbon, a plastic dowel, tape, and tissue paper. They are instructed to develop a plan for making a balloon centerpiece that is stable (not wobbly) and tethers the Mylar helium balloon to the rest of the piece (not floating away). The facilitator supports them in their design work and gives them cues and clues for important steps and considerations. For example, each group needs to consider how they will weigh down the structure appropriately (e.g., putting some small weights or flour or sand in a few balloons at the base). The group also has to consider how to incorporate the dowel or stick into the design so that it provides enough overall support. Students are encouraged to use online resources to help them with planning, problem solving, and adapting appropriately based on the supplies that were provided to them in this group challenge.
MATERIALS	• Inflated Mylar helium balloons • Random assortment of balloons (size/color; make sure there are enough and to properly assess risk for choking) • Tape • Curling ribbon • Tissue paper • A dowel or plastic balloon cup and stick holder
MESSY FACTOR	Low to medium
PINTEREST TERMS	Balloon centerpiece, balloon art, simple balloon weight, balloon garland strategies
GRADE LEVEL	Middle and high schools

essing the Group: Tip Sheet

troduction and Warm-Up Ideas

cuss the differences between being **centered and grounded**

ke a list of occupations that help with being **centered and grounded**; see which ones can be done easily

chool

ays to Grade or Modify the Activity

ovide students with a centerpiece template

ovide more helium balloons that have to be grounded

ke one centerpiece as a group

uestions You May Want to Ask

what ways did the group successfully adapt their design or process once you started building the center-

ce? How do those strategies help with being more **centered and grounded** at school?

hat changes would you expect to see if you could be more **centered and grounded** at school?

hat activities do you tend to neglect when you are not **centered and grounded**?

hat parts of your current routine are helping to stay **centered and grounded**? What changes do you see

ssible for yourself to become more **centered and grounded**?

is was probably a novel activity for you and it certainly had some challenges because of the limited supplies

d directions. Did you find your process for approaching new challenges to be helpful? What might you

ange the next time you have to attempt something challenging?

acilitation Strategies

ncourage students to share adaptive strategies and good ideas with the other groups

onsider having templates ready; remember you want all the groups to experience success

ave some extra supplies in case a balloon pops or determine how you will intentionally process that dimen-

on of the experience

iscuss strategies for building routines at school that offer **centering and grounding** occupations

iscuss the importance of stable and supportive environments on developing habits and routines

Facilitator's Notes

- Successful adaptive strategies (good accommodations and benefits)

- Ways that occupations were discussed to offer **centering and grounding**

- Occupational outcomes that are experienced when one is not **centered and grounded**

- Activities and occupations that would be easy to incorporate into one's routine at school

Group #7

Theresa Carlson Carroll, OTD, OTR/L

GROUP TITLE	Be Your-**selfie** at School
ACTIVITY	Photography
PURPOSE	The purpose of this group is to support students in identifying strengths and developing self-confidence. Students create a visual representation of their strengths, passions, and areas of interest to share with peers. The group fosters self-acceptance and pride and explores options to be one's authentic **selfie** within the school community. Moreover, the group invites participants to consider how occupations are a key way to express one's authentic self. This therapeutic group may be used to working students who are languishing and may tend to have positive screen results for: • Low self-esteem • Judging oneself too harshly • Expects negative reactions or consequences • Difficulty identifying personal strengths or interests • Feels disconnected personally from school • Has difficulty fitting in with others at school • Limited sense of belonging at school • Disinterest in going to school

Be Your-selfie

SESSION GOALS	1. Take several selfies at school that capture images related to a student's person[al] interests, values, and talents.
	2. Work with a partner to arrange the environment to enable certain poses or sh[ots]
	3. Discuss how thinking traps (e.g., paying attention to only negative consequenc[es], being unfairly self-critical, catastrophizing) may impact confidence, how one views themselves, and how one connects with different members of the scho[ol] community.
	4. Make a plan for how to incorporate different personally meaningful activities into the school day to support new habits of thinking that appraise skills more accurately and increase comfort being **oneselfie**.
OCCUPATION AS MEANS AND ENDS	This group uses the occupation of photography to take images of personal strengt[hs] and important aspects of one's occupational identity. The group uses these photos and the experience to explore how access to personally meaningful activities coul[d] help increase self-confidence, self-acceptance, and a positive outlook on going to school.
DIRECTIONS	During this group, students take photos around the school environment to capture images of personal interests, strengths, and values. They work with others to set up the environment and stage the photos. After the photos are taken, participants are encouraged to share images and stories with other group members.
MATERIALS	• Digital cameras • Posterboard to make props and signs • Projector or way to view images
MESSY FACTOR	Low
PINTEREST TERMS	Selfie frames, selfie captions, selfie ideas, selfie ideas creative
GRADE LEVEL	High school but easily adapted for elementary and middle schools

essing the Group: Tip Sheet

Introduction and Warm-Up Ideas

Ask students to share their favorite part of the school day and how they feel during that class, activity, or time

Ask students to imagine a newspaper article is being written about them. What would the title be? What pictures would accompany the article? What would the article be about?

Have students complete a Mad Libs activity about themselves and share with the group if comfortable

Ways to Grade or Modify the Activity

Have props available

Allow participants to draw pictures instead of taking photos

Questions You May Want to Ask

What skills do you notice most when you engage in activities that reflect your interests and are personally meaningful to you?

How do these images reflect what you care deeply about or what matters to you?

How can one use their personal interests to connect with other individuals?

What kinds of goals do you see yourself achieving if you had other people supporting you?

How would you describe the relationship between being able to do the things that you enjoy and your sense of well-being?

What would have to change at school for you to feel more comfortable being yourself?

What are you the proudest of?

What activities would you say you are good enough at?

How did this activity fit with previous experiences you have had at school? How was it different?

Facilitation Strategies

Leverage the social environment to build connection by asking group members to encourage each other and identify ways that members of the group share common interests, feelings, and goals

Be open to exploring environmental barriers at school that may be perceived as barriers to feeling comfortable being oneself, access to activities related to students' personal interests, and so on

Facilitator's Notes

- Personal strengths that were discussed

- Activities that could be incorporated into the school experience that reinforce personal strengths

- Environmental barriers and possible ways to adapt

- How interpersonal dynamics were effective in building connection and discussion among group mem

Group #8

Gina Rainelli, OTD, OTR/L

GROUP TITLE	Making Good Impressions
ACTIVITY	Fabric stamping
PURPOSE	The primary purpose for this fabric stamping craft is to help students strategize how they may begin to rethink activity and behavior choices at school that have not left a good impression. This textile craft occupation challenges students to express their creativity and problem solving to create a unique fabric print using stamps made from things that are good for you—fruits and vegetables! The stamps and patterns should reflect attributes that the student identifies as personal strengths, behavior changes they want to commit to, and choices they wish to make at school. Specifically, students are supported in developing strategies for **stamping out a good impression**.

The group may be helpful for students who present with externalizing behaviors and the following occupational issues:

- Have difficulty making friends
- Participate in bullying others
- Experience social exclusion within the school community
- Experience challenges following school behavioral policies

SESSION GOALS	1. Cut vegetables and fruits to create stamps.
	2. Use the stamps and paint to create a unique textile (e.g., banner or pennant).
	3. Explain how the textile visually represents a plan for changing behaviors and choices at school that will leave a **positive impression** on the school community.

OCCUPATION AS MEANS AND ENDS	This Tier 2 group uses a fabric textile craft to encourage students to develop a plan creating new habits and patterns of behavior that will lead to making better activit choices and meeting student role expectations.
DIRECTIONS	This group activity primarily focuses on creating banners/pennants to hang in the school's physical environment to support students in rethinking ways they can reframe their identity and influence on the social environment at school. Students use their creativity to create patterns from vegetables and fabric paint to stamp ou their commitment to upholding the school and classroom rules and participating in activities that are consistent with the school environment. They discuss personal strengths and talents that will likely become more apparent to others if they are successful in **stamping out a good impression**. Additionally, they discuss how different occupational and activity choices could change people's impression of th to a more favorable one.
MATERIALS	• Vegetables and fruits (e.g., apples, green pepper, carrots, potato, mushrooms, f broccoli, celery) • Knife to cut fruits and vegetables • Cookie cutters • Fabric paint • Fabric pens (to write words and quotes) • Pie tins or paper plates for the paint • Felt, fabric squares, or pennants • Sponges or sponge brushes to spread the paint on the vegetables and fruit • Puffy paint or fabric pens to write antibullying messages • Fine-point markers to add detail • Paper towels and cleaning solution or wipes for clean-up • Paper to cover the table
MESSY FACTOR	High
PINTEREST TERMS	Veggie stamps, fun ways to stamp with your veggies, DIY potato print textiles, uniqu veggie fabric prints, personalized pennant, pennant flags DIY, felt pennants
GRADE LEVEL	Middle school

k Vegetable and Fruit Stamp Tip Sheet

able or Fruit	Design Ideas
	Small flowers
n the cob	Rain drops, seeds
pepper	Shamrock
of celery stems	Roses
	Butterfly
ower	Brain
oom	Brain
	Snails, coils, maze
	Carve out many different shapes

essing the Group: Tip Sheet

troduction and Warm-Up Ideas

ive the group brainstorm unconventional or novel ways that one could use a paperclip (or another com-
on object) to prepare them for the unconventional use of the vegetables and fruits

ays to Grade or Modify the Activity

ecut and preprint materials

ovide examples of stamping patterns and designs to help brainstorming

onsider a placemat instead of a pennant

ake stamps from other kinds of materials (foam, soaps, erasers)

se paper or cardboard instead of felt

uestions You May Want to Ask

you had opportunities to use your skills and abilities at school more frequently, what kinds of hidden tal-
ts would people uncover?

hat kinds of activities can support you in developing a habit around making behavioral choices that are
ore consistent with school rules?

hat do you want your legacy or lasting impression to be on the school? What changes are needed for that to happen?

ow might the strategies you used to turn vegetables into stamps be useful when turning a bad impression
to a **positive or good impression**?

he pennant you made will provide you with a nice reminder of your commitment to make changes. What
ther ways could the environment be used to provide support or cues?

hat resources or supports will you need to fulfill this commitment?

hat new habits will be helpful in making a **new and positive impression**?

acilitation Strategies

e sure to go over safety rules and expectations for using knife or carving tools

upport self-efficacy by identifying and sharing your observations of skills they are using well as they work
n different parts of the project

ncourage language that reflects a commitment to change

ake links between the actions one takes and the impression(s) left behind

Facilitator's Notes

- Change talk that represents commitment (desire to change, reasons to change)

- Ways to leverage the environment to increase support for change

- New or more adaptive habits and expectations for how impressions shift

Group #9

Christine Kivlen, PhD, OTR/L
and Jenna L. Heffron, PhD, OTR/L

GROUP TITLE	Spreading Our Wings: Caterpillars to CAN-DO-pillars
ACTIVITY	Daily journaling and origami
	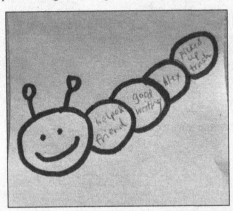 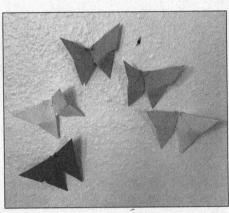
PURPOSE	The purpose of this therapeutic group is to explore how students can develop confidence in being able to ask for support and access to activities that use their skills and talents at school. The group primarily supports a short daily check-in/check-out group that challenges students to recognize and reflect on activity choices, how personal skills were used, and actions taken to be a positive member of the classroom and school community.

The purpose of this therapeutic group is to explore how students can develop confidence in being able to ask for support and access to activities that use their skills and talents at school. The group primarily supports a short daily check-in/check-out group that challenges students to recognize and reflect on activity choices, how personal skills were used, and actions taken to be a positive member of the classroom and school community.

This activity is envisioned to be part of a small group check-in/check-out program to support learners to increase motivation for school occupations through building self-esteem, self-awareness, and self-determination. Each morning, students pick up their daily sticky note containing a caterpillar drawing and prompts along different body segments. Students are directed to transform their caterpillar into a **CAN-DO-pillar** by placing an "X" in each body segment that reflects something they **can do** at school. At the end of the day, students meet briefly to check out how well they addressed the prompts. If all prompts were addressed, then they are invited to turn their sticky note into a butterfly and add it to the wall of butterflies mural.

This Tier 2 small group may be most useful to students who have positive screens and occupational issues related to:

- Feeling overwhelmed by challenges at school
- Effectively solving mundane challenges at school
- Lacking self-esteem to confidently interact with peers
- Having a limited sense of skill and preference for tasks that are easy
- Asking for what they need to perform and participate fully in school situations and tasks

SESSION GOALS	1. Orient students to the check-in/check-out process over the next few weeks.
	2. Go over the mini sticky note journals and how to fill in the caterpillar.
	3. Teach and practice making an origami butterfly from the sticky note.
	4. Show pictures or describe how all the origami butterflies come together to ma[ke] a big mural in the school.
OCCUPATION AS MEANS AND ENDS	This therapeutic group uses a modified daily journaling activity to support habit training to build self-confidence and strengthen self-determination at school.
DIRECTIONS	The group session provides students with an overview of the modified daily journa[l] using sticky notes and an opportunity to practice filling in one entry. Each sticky n[ote] will have four prompts or affirmations located on segments of the caterpillar's body "I can make good choices that are right for me at school today!", "I can use my skills at school today!", "I can ask for help if I need it!", and "I can be a positive member of my school community today!" Students are asked to minimally put an "X" on each segment of the caterpillar's body to identify something they **can do**. Students try t[o] put an "X" on each segment to turn the caterpillar into a **CAN-DO-pillar**. Students are strongly encouraged to write down key words or details highlighting situations [or] experiences that reinforce what they **can do** at school, which will be shared during the check-out meeting. Students also practice transforming the sticky note into a butterfly according to simple origami directions. Several attempts to practice the origami folds are likely to be needed.
	During the daily check-in activity, each group member is given a sticky note with a caterpillar and discusses plans for approaching the day positively. They are reminde[d] to jot down examples of how they are following the prompts. During the check-ou[t] activity at the end of the school day, the students share how they transformed thei[r] caterpillar into a **CAN-DO-pillar**. Then they transform their sticky notes into origam[i] butterflies, which will be featured prominently in the school environment to reinfor[ce] their progress!
MATERIALS	• Preprinted sticky notes • Origami butterfly instructions • Pencil or pen
MESSY FACTOR	Low
PINTEREST TERMS	Easy origami butterfly, kids origami, origami ideas for beginners, basic origami butterfly
GRADE LEVEL	Late elementary and middle schools

essing the Group: Tip Sheet

troduction and Warm-Up Ideas

ctice making origami butterflies from sticky notes

ok at different pictures of origami butterfly murals so they can anticipate how their daily contributions will
ve a bigger picture

ays to Grade or Modify the Activity

ve students a step-by-step origami butterfly handout

crease the number of **can do** prompts that need to be completed each day at school

ainstorm activity ideas with a student if they are unable to address all the prompts

uestions You May Want to Ask

ow do you imagine you can transform yourself at school in ways similar to how origami helps transform
e paper into a butterfly? What resources will you need?

hat kinds of environments are most comfortable for you to ask for help in? How could the school environ-
ent be changed or modified to make it more comfortable to ask for help?

ho do you feel comfortable asking for help? How do they help you at school?

hat kinds of things can you achieve at school if you had more opportunities to use your skills and talents?

hat are the aspects of school that you **can do** well at?

ow do you imagine school will be if you practice doing all of the prompts: "I can make good choices that
e right for me at school today!", "I can use my skills at school today!", "I can ask for help if I need it!", and "I
n be a positive member of my school community today!"

ow might an increase in confidence be helpful in feeling connected with other people at school (e.g., friends,
achers, staff)?

acilitation Strategies

o not impose any punishments on students who do not address all daily prompts; simply encourage them
complete the daily journal note the next day

elp them to understand the importance of daily work to build new habits

Facilitator's Notes

- What students noted they **can do** easily

- What activities can build/strengthen self-confidence

- How praise was offered to reinforce errorless learning

Group #10

Ashley Hettlinger, MSOT, OTR/L
and Susan Cahill, PhD, OTR/L, FAOTA

GROUP TITLE	Juggling It All
ACTIVITY	Juggling
PURPOSE	The purpose of this group activity is to support students in understanding that **juggling** occupational demands is essential to meeting the expectations of different roles at school. This therapeutic group introduces a process and time to practice juggling three (or more) scarves. Students are invited to explore strategies and ways to reconfigure their processes for **juggling** different aspects of being a student. This Tier 2 group may be helpful to students who present with occupational concerns at school and whose screens reveal the following difficulties: • Managing multiple role demands at school • Worrying about over-commitment or over-involvement in relation to school and extracurricular activities • Organizing time use efficiently • Balancing academic obligations and other responsibilities
SESSION GOALS	1. Try to **juggle** at least three scarves. 2. Make a list of what strategies and methods seem to produce the best effects. 3. Make a list of skills used for **juggling**. 4. Apply the metaphor to issues at school that have been hard for them to **juggle**.
OCCUPATION AS MEANS AND ENDS	This group uses the occupation of juggling to explore occupational competence and the student's ability more deeply to "**juggle**" and meet expectations associated with multiple roles (e.g., friend, peer, student, classmate, group member).

DIRECTIONS	During this group, students learn how to juggle three scarves at a time by either watching videos or being provided by a demonstration. Students are encouraged work up to juggling three scarves at the same time. Students will:
	<ul><li>Select three scarves of different colors</li><li>Practice the cross and throw motion with one scarf until they feel comfortable</li><li>Add in scarf two when comfortable</li><li>Progress to the third scarf</li><li>Continue practicing and make as much progress as they can</li></ul>After students have been given time to practice their juggling skills, the second ph of the group focuses on applying their actual experiences of juggling scarves to th current experiences of feeling overwhelmed trying to **juggle everything at schoc** To process the group, students will:<ul><li>Reflect on their current roles (e.g., student, family member, athlete, club memb and the demands associated with each</li><li>Compare the strategies and skills needed to juggle the scarves to the strategie: needed to **juggle everything at school**</li><li>Consider if there are any roles or occupations that could be or need to be "dropped"</li></ul>
MATERIALS	<ul><li>Three different colored nylon scarves for each participant (or fewer sets of scarv if students take turns juggling)</li><li>Demonstration or video</li></ul>
MESSY FACTOR	Low
PINTEREST TERMS	Activity scarves, easy-to-use juggling scarves, scarf activities
GRADE LEVEL	Middle school

essing the Group: Tip Sheet

troduction and Warm-Up Ideas

ovide an opportunity to play with the scarves and juggle before showing a video or giving instructions

ther their opinions on juggling (Do they think it is easy or hard? Do they already know how to juggle? This

uld be helpful information for the facilitator.)

ays to Grade or Modify the Activity

o-ball juggling

y to keep a few balloons in the air as a team (if juggling is too hard)

courage them to try more challenging patterns

fferent objects (e.g., ping pong balls, sock balls)

onsider spreading the group over multiple sessions

uestions You May Want to Ask

hat skills helped you be successful in juggling today? How might those skills help you become better at **ggling** your responsibilities at school?

hat changes in your performance would make you proud of yourself? Did today's activity help you identify mething you can change?

what ways did you expect that you would juggle successfully? Or in what ways were you surprised by your ility to juggle well?

hat did you observe when scarves or objects fell to the ground? How do you normally approach situations school when it is just too hard to **juggle** and keep everything in the air? Did this activity offer any new oughts on what you may want to do the next time?

hat responsibilities at school are the most important to you?

acilitation Strategies

ormalize that juggling is difficult literally and metaphorically

elp them to explore ways the social environment may also be leveraged and how other people can some-mes help us keep things in the air while we reset

vite them to identify a change they feel confident making soon and encourage them to commit to taking a ew approach by saying it out loud

Facilitator's Notes

- What skills students reported

- Offer them ways to see they are doing better than they anticipated

- Make lists of observations visible to support processing

- Suggest differences between feeling like you have to **juggle everything yourself** vs. using the environm either help you **juggle** or to provide a secure space to set things for future use

- Responses to things dropping

Group #11

Brad E. Egan, OTD, PhD, CADC, OTR/L
and Stephanie Brauch, MSOT, OTR/L

GROUP TITLE	When Connection Seems Difficult: A Paper Chain Tapestry
ACTIVITY	Paper chains/wall hanging
	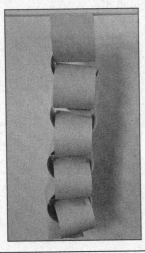 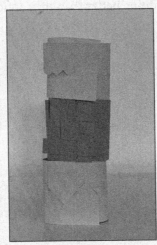 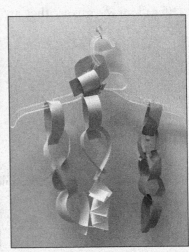
PURPOSE	The purpose of this therapeutic group activity is to provide students with an opportunity to consider alternative strategies for connecting with members of their school community. Students who feel connected to others at school and accepted for who they are look forward to going to school. Connection is a critical factor that supports mental well-being at school. Occupations may serve as a means for building connections and/or developing ways to practice new strategies.
	During the activity, group members are challenged to create a paper chain tapestry together. To support creative problem solving and reflection around difficulties connecting to others at school, participants are provided with any adhesive or binding materials (e.g., glue, tape, staples). Using only scissors, group members have to figure out how to connect the paper chains, which can be accomplished fairly simply by cutting and folding. Moreover, group members are encouraged to consider a design or pattern that links the individual paper chain strands together. Participants are invited to reflect during the group on parallels between how they experience the **difficulties connecting** the paper chains and the **difficulties connecting** to members of the school community.

	This group may be helpful to students who experience the following occupationa[l] issues at school: • Seem to be withdrawn or apathetic owing to difficulty collaborating and cooperating with peers and/or teachers on shared problems • Difficulty initiating or maintaining friendships with individuals or groups of frie[nds] • Poor resiliency with new or unexpected assignments, circumstances, or encounters that may present as disinterest or apathy • Do not contribute to group or class assignments or discussions owing to inabil[ity] to recognize their own strengths and contributions
SESSION GOALS	1. Create paper chains without any traditional adhesive supplies. 2. Evaluate the strategies for connecting without adhesive supplies. 3. Consider how the activity parallels their experiences trying to connect with oth[er] people at school. 4. Consider how the strategies used in the activity may apply to school situations[.]
OCCUPATION AS MEANS AND ENDS	This therapeutic group uses an art/craft project to assist students in identifying alternative strategies for connecting with other peers and staff members in the sch[ool] community.
DIRECTIONS	Group members are presented with a stack of different colored paper, two pairs of scissors, and a clothes hanger. They are asked to make a paper chain wall tapestry b[y] connecting and hanging individual chains from the hanger. During the first phase, they try to problem solve how they can connect each link and chains without any adhesive or binding materials. The occupational therapy facilitator may offer differe[nt] support strategies and hints. Once they develop a strategy, the group is tasked with trying to create a pattern that incorporates and connects each strand of paper links[.]
MATERIALS	• Several pieces of construction paper (can be various colors and patterns) • Two pairs of scissors • A plastic or wooden clothes hanger or tapestry hanger • Art supplies (to decorate paper and create pattern)
MESSY FACTOR	Low
PINTEREST TERMS	Paper chain craft, paper garland, paper chain wall art, paper chain wall hanging
GRADE LEVEL	Middle and high schools

essing the Group: Tip Sheet

troduction and Warm-Up Ideas

eate a small dot-to-dot pattern without instructions; this should quickly jump-start a conversation about **ficulties connecting** the dots

ke a list of some of the barriers they discuss

ays to Grade or Modify the Activity

ovide the group with a template that easily enables connecting chains without any adhesive materials

courage the group to consider a design for the wall hanging

e white paper and add a design after the paper chains have been placed on the hanger

uestions You May Want to Ask

ow might connections develop from participating in activities that align with shared personal interests and lues?

hat skills support you in learning about what others are interested in?

hat skills do you consider to be the most needed to connect with other people?

hich places and spaces at school are easier to interact in? Which places and spaces are more challenging to teract in?

hat strategy helped you to accomplish the goal of connecting the paper chains in this activity? How might u use that same strategy when trying to connect with other people at school?

id you expect that you would be able to connect the paper chains together without glue or tape? Do you pically expect that you will be successful in connecting with other people at school?

ow well would you say that you performed at making connections in this activity?

you develop new strategies for connecting, like you discovered in this activity, what kinds of school activi- es do you think will be easier to participate in?

hat aspects of this activity, if any, did you relate to the most?

acilitation Strategies

ncourage students to brainstorm strategies together

onsider allowing students to search online for ideas

einforce the value of trying new approaches to solve ongoing challenges

emonstrate one approach to connecting the paper without tape or glue if the group struggles

Facilitator's Notes

- Students' motivation to work through a challenge

- Different strategies that were used (those that were successful vs. those that did not work out)

- Any resources used

- How group members supported each other during the activity and discussion

- The parallels between having to problem solve and making connections in a difficult context with chains and with others at school

Group #12

Caitlin Esposito, OTD, OTR/L

GROUP TITLE	What I Bring to the Table
ACTIVITY	Pizza topping art
PURPOSE	The primary purpose for this creative cooking activity is to create an opportunity for students to identify positive characteristics they recognize in themselves. The group invites them to do so by making designs with pizza toppings to self-identify strengths and talents and to share with everyone what they **bring to the table**. Students in this Tier 2 group discuss the barriers and opportunities that exist at school for bringing those skills and talents to the table. They also identify ways they may be able to combine their skills and talents with academic work and projects to make going to school more enjoyable. The concept of what they **bring to the table** is also discussed in terms of planning for their future after high school.

Understanding and using one's skills and talents in daily activities is necessary for finding meaning and experiencing personal satisfaction from one's daily routine. When students struggle integrating their skills and talents with academic work, school can become boring and be a source of dread. It may become challenging to adopt academic goals, participate in student role/school tasks, or desire school success the more a student sees school as being disconnected from the meaningful aspects of their daily life. **Bringing personal strengths and talents to the table** when doing academic tasks may be a useful way to increase a student's motivation to participate in school activities.

The group may be helpful for students who are languishing personally and may tend to:

- Have difficulty recognizing personal strengths
- Be unsure of what they figuratively **bring to the table**
- Make self-deprecating comments
- Lack a sense of belonging to the greater school community
- Perceive school as boring or unfulfilling
- Have difficulty or have stopped including school tasks into their routine

SESSION GOALS	1. Explore personal strengths. 2. Decide on designs that represent strengths, unique qualities, and distinct thing the student **brings to the table**. 3. Create designs using pizza toppings. 4. Have a pizza party and process the activity.
OCCUPATION AS MEANS AND ENDS	This group uses the occupation of cooking, specifically pizza, to explore self-identif strengths and talents. As an ends, students identify ways they may be able to use what they **bring to the table** to experience greater satisfaction from their school experiences.
DIRECTIONS	Students create an individual pizza using different toppings to create a design that metaphorically represents their personal strengths and talents that could be better integrated into their approach to school. Students have a few minutes to sketch a design and consider the different available toppings. Then, they translate the desig onto small pizzas using the toppings and bake according to directions. Before eatin their completed products, students share with the group what they **bring to the table** by describing their individual design. Moreover, the group discusses strategie to bring their skills and talents to the table more easily and what the likely effect wi be on their current levels of participation and satisfaction as a student.
MATERIALS	• Store-bought pizza dough or individual crusts for each member • Pizza sauce • Variety of pizza toppings (cheese, pepperoni, sausage, onions, green peppers, black olives, ham, pineapple, chicken, banana peppers, spinach, mushrooms, etc • Pizza pans for baking • Parchment paper to line pizza pan • Oven or cooking appliance • Sink for washing dishes • One pair of gloves for each participant • Pizza cutter or knife for facilitator to use when pizzas are done
MESSY FACTOR	High
PINTEREST TERMS	Yummy pizza art, DIY superhero pizza, impressive pizza art, smiling face pizza
GRADE LEVEL	High school

essing the Group: Tip Sheet

troduction and Warm-Up Ideas
ve students generate a list of words that describe them and then do an image search

ays to Grade or Modify the Activity
corate prebaked cookies to eliminate need for an oven and baking
ke English muffin or bagel pizzas

uestions You May Want to Ask
hat personal strengths or characteristics are you most proud of?
hat skills have been challenging for you to demonstrate in school tasks?
hat settings make it easier for you to **bring your talents and skills to the table**? In what ways could the
1ool environment be changed to make this easier for you?
ow do you see what you **bring to the table** influencing your future goals positively?
ow might the skills you **bring to the table** support you in handling your school tasks and responsibilities
tter?
iis activity hopefully reminded you of some strengths and positive things you **bring to the table**. What
her activities are you good at? How might you go about including those into your routine more often?

acilitation Strategies
icourage group members to acknowledge strengths and talents that each other **brings to the table**
ipport self-efficacy by allowing them to problem solve solutions they feel may work for them
onsider interventions that target the school environment based on barriers and experiences shared

Facilitator's Notes

- What the students reported in terms of skills

- Sources of dissatisfaction

- Changes and expectations for making changes

- Encourage the possibility to consider how different activity choices could enable more satisfaction with to school

Group #13

*Ryan Thomure, OTD, OTR/L, LCSW
and Ray Cendejas, COTA/L*

GROUP TITLE	The Building Blocks of the Day
ACTIVITY	Game
PURPOSE	Students who struggle to manage a stable and satisfying routine are less skillful at balancing the demands of school alongside extracurricular activities, family obligations, and other tasks without sacrificing strong academic performance. This group uses a wooden block tower game to explore the literal parallels between approaching an increasingly more unstable tower and navigating school responsibilities with an increasingly more unstable daily routine. Students are also encouraged to explore the different factors that appear to be most responsible for recent destabilizing shifts with respect to meeting student role expectations. The group may be helpful for students who are experiencing occupational concerns associated with: • Struggling with school–life balance • Feeling overwhelmed at school • Feeling large amount of stress at school • Not being able to effectively organize their schedule • Poor adherence to homework or other assignments • Difficulty handling multiple responsibilities

SESSION GOALS	1. Play several rounds of the game.
	2. Intentionally reflect on the overall stability of the structure at different points ir the game.
	3. Consider ways to make changes to one's school routine.
OCCUPATION AS MEANS AND ENDS	This group uses a wooden block tower game to explore the literal parallels associat with removing blocks and creating an increasingly more unstable tower and sustaining a daily routine in the presence of factors that contribute to occupational imbalance, especially with respect to school occupations and student roles.
DIRECTIONS	The tower consists of 39 or more wooden blocks stacked in alternating stories of th blocks. Players attempt to dismantle the tower by using one hand to skillfully remo a block from the tower and place it on the top story. Players may elect to remove a block below the highest completed story. It may be helpful to test how loose a blo may be. However, if the player shifts the position of the block, they must use one hand to return it to its original position without causing the tower to tumble before selecting another block. The goal is not to be the player who causes the tower to topple over in whole or in part. The winner of the game is the last player who adde piece to the tower before it toppled. Players should allow for there to be at least 5 seconds between turns to make sure the tower is stable and not going to fall ove
MATERIALS	• Tower block building game • Deck of cards (warm-up activity) • Whiteboard and markers for discussion
MESSY FACTOR	Low to medium
PINTEREST TERMS	Wooden tower game, toppling tower, stacking tower, giant yard tower, soda box tov
GRADE LEVEL	High school

essing the Group: Tip Sheet

troduction and Warm-Up Ideas

ve individuals try to make a simple tower of cards (approximately 10 cards)

amine the stability of each structure and their relative confidence that their structure could withstand ce/pressure

ays to Grade or Modify the Activity

ay with life-size blocks (empty boxes/12-pack soda boxes)

corporate different forces (wind from fan, moving surface) to explore how the environment may also im-ct stability

uestions You May Want to Ask

hat does a balanced day look like for you?

hat skills and coping strategies have you used in the past to pick up the pieces or rebuild after parts of your e have become unstable or fell apart like the tower? How might you use those skills to add some stability your life now?

what ways does a routine offer a sense of stability? What changes might you be open to considering that uld create more stability in your life?

hat kinds of places and spaces make you feel most stable and in control?

ow do important relationships impact your sense of control and stability?

what ways do you feel this activity represents your current experiences?

hat habits or approaches have caused the most instability? What new habits or approaches could add stabil-y to your life?

hat will you need to implement those new habits successfully at school?

acilitation Strategies

rite their reactions and quotes down as they play the game

upport self-efficacy by identifying and sharing your observations of skills they are using well as they work n different parts of the project

elp to manage the daily task list so you can monitor how students handle responsibilities

Facilitator's Notes

- Issues that are causing imbalances

- Environment factors that provide stability

- Strategies to modify routine

- New habits identified

Group #14

*Patricia (Patee) Tomsic, OTD, MS, OTR/L
and Anthony (Tony) Mesiano, Jr., MSW, LCSW, BCD, NCAC-1*

OUP TITLE	Escape to Zen
TIVITY	Escape room and zendoodle
RPOSE	The purpose of this group is to provide students with an opportunity to engage in a mindful activity at school. This therapeutic group uses a simple escape room game and a zendoodling art project to assist students in identifying activities that can be done at school to help them experience increased calm and self-control to better adapt to stressful situations and perform social interaction skills more effectively during exchanges with peers and staff. Additionally, the zendoodle activity uses an errorless activity framework so all participants are successful.

The purpose of this group is to provide students with an opportunity to engage in a mindful activity at school. This therapeutic group uses a simple escape room game and a zendoodling art project to assist students in identifying activities that can be done at school to help them experience increased calm and self-control to better adapt to stressful situations and perform social interaction skills more effectively during exchanges with peers and staff. Additionally, the zendoodle activity uses an errorless activity framework so all participants are successful.

Many students with externalizing behaviors may benefit from intentional participation in activities that promote mindfulness during the day. Occupational therapy practitioners can support students in developing habits associated with mindfulness and building school routines that pre-emptively incorporate mindfulness activities so they feel greater control when completing school tasks.

This group may be helpful to students who:

- Get in trouble for acting out
- Present with externalizing behaviors when asked to collaborate or cooperate with peers and/or teachers
- Have difficulty initiating or maintaining friendships with individuals or groups of friends
- Exhibit poor resiliency with new or unexpected circumstances at school
- Exhibit poor coping
- Do not contribute to group or class assignments or discussions owing to inability to recognize their own strengths and contributions

SESSION GOALS	1. Complete the escape challenge to get the directions for zendoodling. 2. Discuss being mindful vs. mindless. 3. Complete a zendoodle mindfully.
OCCUPATION AS MEANS AND ENDS	A simple escape room game and a zendoodling art project are used to help stude identify activities that can be done at school to promote adaptation to stressful situations.
DIRECTIONS	This group is divided into two phases. **Phase 1:** Students work in a small group to complete a quick escape room exercise The forms have been provided to make set-up simple. Participants should proceed through the escape room challenge in this order: read the diary entries, find the key unlock the padlock on the scissors, and use the scissors to cut the balloon and retri the final clue—instructions on zendoodling. **Phase 2:** Group participants follow the instructions for how to zendoodle. The occupational therapy facilitator reinforces the errorless framework to ensure all participants know there is no right or wrong in zendoodling. The occupational ther facilitator encourages repetitive doodling to support deeper levels of mindfulness. Students share their doodles with one another and discuss to what extent they reached a sense of calm while zendoodling.
MATERIALS	• A blank notebook to serve as the diary • Printed diary entries (provided) • Optional clue (provided) • A padlock with a key • Envelope • Tape • Balloons • Printed zendoodle instructions • Paper • Pens • Colored pencils
MESSY FACTOR	Low
PINTEREST TERMS	Breakout challenge, easy escape room ideas, zendoodle
GRADE LEVEL	Middle school (as written) and high school (make challenges more difficult)

essing the Group: Tip Sheet

troduction and Warm-Up Ideas

ovide descriptions and definitions of breakout challenges, breakout boxes, and/or escape rooms to educate
ose who may be unfamiliar with the task

k students to think of activities in which they have experienced flow or felt a momentary escape to being
the zone

cape room activity can essentially serve as the warm-up

ays to Grade or Modify the Activity

e coloring or another activity to support mindfulness

ake the escape room activities more challenging for older students

quire the zendoodles be turned in for a final clue

uestions You May Want to Ask

hat activities/occupations are most helpful in providing a **temporary escape**? How does taking **temporary
capes** support our mental well-being or **feeling zen at school**?

hat skills were you aware of when you were trying to doodle mindfully and complete your **zendoodle**?

hat would it look like for you if you were intentional about doing mindful activities throughout the school
y to provide yourself with **temporary escapes** and restoration?

ow might participating in mindful activities help you to decrease other behaviors that are interfering with
ing able to follow school rules or meet others' expectations?

here is no right or wrong in a zendoodle. What did you notice about your performance since that expecta-
on was removed? What impact does the pressure to be right (not be wrong) have on your performance at
hool?

hat effect does **feeling zen** have on your ability to think before you act? On your ability to make choices
at align with your goals?

hat would the school day look like if you no longer felt the need to try and **mentally escape** it?

hat did you experience in this group activity or discuss that may help you cope or behave in ways that are
ore consistent with school rules?

acilitation Strategies

his group requires some preparation time for the escape room challenges to go smoothly, so the following
rder is suggested: (1) Glue the provided diary entries into a notebook with the word "diary" written on the
over; (2) glue an envelope to the back of the notebook and place the key to unlock the padlock in it; (3) roll
p the zendoodle instructions and place them in the balloon before inflating and tying a knot; and (4) lock
e scissors using the padlock as shown

ake a list of activities associated with the experience of flow and ask about how often they engage in re-
orted activities

ncourage participants to reflect on their focus and concentration during the activity

onsider having some examples of zendoodle patterns to help them understand the repetitive nature of the
ctivity

Facilitator's Notes

- Issues that have resulted from not thinking before acting

- Examples that distinguish mindfulness from mindlessness

- Impact of occupation or activity on mental well-being

- Skills from observations that are helpful to adapting and coping

r Diary,

as a different kind of day at school yesterday. I had an opportunity to try something
. That doesn't happen very often, so it was a *nice surprise*. I kind of liked it. I was *surprised*
ow well everyone did. I mean all the art **turn**ed out cool.

for now.

---

r Diary,

you ever just wonder how to *calm yourself down*? I mean, sometimes I just wish I had
e activities that I could do at school that would help me *simmer down fast*. I will *keep*
ing for **the** strategy. If I have to spend most of my day there, I'd like to make it as chill as
sible.

er.

---

r Diary,

e you ever heard of a teacher actually teaching kids to put an argument *together*? My
lish teacher actually went **over** how to put a logical argument *together* today. Seemed
d of funny to me since I am usually in trouble for arguing. Maybe **the** issue is in how I do
'm interested to find out more about this. Maybe I have something to learn.

os.

CASE YOU NEED A CLUE!

se people understand that dwelling in the past does not usually provide dividends.
eaming too far into the future can limit your ability to **BOLDLY** be in the present. That is
gift of calm. That is the gift of zen. **Do you see any bolded words?**

Place this clue in the envelope on the back of the diary:

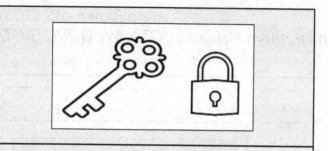

You have found the key! Use this key to unlock the scissors and prepare for an experience designed to make you feel as light as a balloon. **Hint. Hint.**

Place these instructions in the balloon before inflating it. Have a group member read the directions to the s

Congratulations!! You successfully worked through the clues. Are you ready to find some ZEN? For the next activity, try something called zendoodling. Maybe that's a new word, s I'll explain what it is and the steps below.

A zendoodle is an art project designed to bring the artist a sense of calm, a release of stress, and an invitation to be mindful. Get creative! Escape into the activity! There is no right or wrong when it comes to zendoodling—everything works and is okay in a zendoodle!

Steps for zendoodling:

1. Get a pencil or a pen.

2. Draw a square tile roughly 3 inches by 3 inches.

3. Divide your square into several sections by making different bold lines. Consider abou six that run the length or width of the square. Maybe the line is wavy, curvy, or creates loop.

4. Now is the fun part. In each section use your creativity to design a simple repetitive doodle pattern. Try to keep your focus on your pattern. Get into the zen.

5. When your square is full of doodle, consider shading or adding some pops of color.

6. Admire your creative work!

Group #15

Anna Brown, MS, OTR/L
and Kathryn M. Loukas, OTD, MS, OTR/L, FAOTA

GROUP TITLE	Moving Target Practice: Aiming for Success
ACTIVITY	Target practice
PURPOSE	The purpose of this therapeutic group activity is to provide students with an opportunity to explore strategies that can **improve our aim** when dealing with situations that are changing or when it feels like the **targets are moving**. During this activity, students participate in a fun target practice with **moving targets**. They are asked to keep a record of the number of trials and the number of times they hit the bullseye. A running list of strategies that helped **adapt to moving targets** are posted to prompt reflection after the activity.
	Students who adapt well to changing circumstances and uncertainty are able to achieve more academically. They also experience less fear with taking risks and learning from mistakes than students who feel less capable or helpless. They approach uncertainty or change as a potential opportunity to problem solve a challenge, develop a new talent or skill, and learn how to identify situational aspects that may be open to change or require flexibility.
	This Tier 2 group may be helpful for students whose screens reflect occupational challenges associated with:
	• Becoming overwhelmed by changing circumstances at school
	• Feeling helpless
	• Difficulty adapting to change
	• Needing help and support to do things they historically performed well in at school
	• Experience angst and dread when school tasks are less structured
	• Spending energy trying to control situations
	• Expecting negative outcomes when situations are uncertain

SESSION GOALS	1. Try to hit the "X" or bullseye on a moving target.
	2. Name different strategies being used to increase aim for moving targets.
	3. Decide which strategies worked best.
	4. Determine if these strategies can be useful when handling situations at school that are uncertain and may feel like aiming at **moving targets**.
OCCUPATION AS MEANS AND ENDS	This group uses a safe and fun target-throwing game to explore how to develop better habits when participating in situations that have some level of uncertainty a require flexibility at school.
DIRECTIONS	Students are instructed that the object of the game is to hit as many targets as possible. The facilitator marks an "X" or target on each balloon and hangs them from the ceiling using streamer and tape. Students roll up clean socks into balls to throw the targets and are encouraged to try different strategies (e.g., manipulate the size the ball, figure out ways to move the air flow to create less movement, make the "X bigger, create a new boundary line). An oscillating floor fan is used to set the target motion and a target line is set to ensure a certain minimum distance from the targe The rest will be fun, problem solving, and aiming for success.
MATERIALS	• Balloons
	• Marker to draw a target on each balloon
	• Streamers
	• Tape
	• Clean socks
	• Oscillating fan or wind generator
MESSY FACTOR	Low
PINTEREST TERMS	Balloon-moving target, moving color targets, paper plate bullseye, kid's target pract
GRADE LEVEL	Middle school (discuss the importance of not throwing at each other and general safety)

essing the Group: Tip Sheet

troduction and Warm-Up Ideas

ve students roll socks into soft balls that will be used during target practice

ve students mark the "X" (**target**) on the balloons.

k questions about how going to school fits into **aiming for success**

ays to Grade or Modify the Activity

e smaller balls to make it harder or larger balls to make it easier

hange the speed of the moving targets for ease or difficulty

onsider the distance between the student and the target and increase or decrease accordingly

troduce changes in environment, rules of play, or objectives to make the process more uncertain

uestions You May Want to Ask

e had fun playing this game when things were changing and the targets were moving. In what ways was it fferent for you to participate in this activity vs. when you have to participate in activities that are changing school?

hat strategies did you use that **helped you aim at and hit your moving target** better? In what ways could e consider some of these strategies when doing activities that seem to change a lot at school?

u hit your **targets**!! What are some of the **targets** or goals that you have at school? How successful do you ink you will feel when accomplishing those goals? What skills will you use to **hit those targets**?

cture yourself **hitting all your targets** at school. Describe what that day at school would look like. What ould you be proud of? Who would also be cheering you on? What **moving targets** would you have success-lly hit?

itting moving targets can seem really hard, especially when we **miss the target**. But it was easy to pick up e ball and try to **hit the target** again. What things at school do you think you could probably accomplish you committed to trying again?

ased on this group experience, what is one small change you could begin to make that would help your aim d help you **hit some targets** at school?

acilitation Strategies

eep the atmosphere light

ormalize that it is hard to hit the "X" or bullseye

linimize any mistakes or instances when the target was missed

lake a list of the strategies you see them using

Facilitator's Notes

- What strategies helped to hit the moving targets

- How did they change or adapt the environment

- Ways that you kept them motivated to try and **hit the target** after missing

- Examples of how changing circumstances has caused issues at school

Group #16

Ashley Hettlinger, MSOT, OTR/L
and Susan Cahill, PhD, OTR/L, FAOTA

GROUP TITLE	Kaleidoscope of Colors and Change
ACTIVITY	Craft
PURPOSE	The purpose of this activity is to help students understand that not all change is bad. Change is a part of everyday life and can often be positive. During this activity, the students make a kaleidoscope and examine the images it creates from various perspectives. The changing image in the kaleidoscope is used as a metaphor to explore the changes each student experiences. Group members discuss how they have experienced and coped with change in their own lives and at school. This Tier 2 small group intervention may be helpful for students who are: • Feeling overwhelmed by the changes brought about by regular transitions from one grade or learning environment to the next • Experiencing a life event that leads to change (e.g., parental divorce, parent losing a job, moving to a new school) • Avoiding new experiences (i.e., lack of flexibility) • Having difficulty using strengths and abilities to cope
SESSION GOALS	1. Each group member makes a personal kaleidoscope. 2. Discuss current thoughts about a personal change affecting school. 3. Identify potentially new perspectives to consider.

OCCUPATION AS MEANS AND ENDS	Students make a craft that provides opportunities to view ever-changing patterns consider possibilities for developing new ways of thinking about change and habit support coping when situations may change.
DIRECTIONS	During this group, students construct a kaleidoscope and discuss the habit of view the changes caused by transition from multiple perspectives. Students will: • Construct and decorate a kaleidoscope • Reflect on how their frame changes • Consider how changes would be viewed from multiple perspectives • Practice the habit of thinking about change from multiple perspectives
MATERIALS	• Paper towel tube (or piece of wrapping paper tube) • 12 inches by 12 inches cardstock • Thin, clear plastic (can be scrap) • Colorful beads • Sequins • Cardboard • Aluminum foil • Scissors • Hot glue gun • Markers • Rubber bands • Washi tape or stickers (or other decorations for the tube)
MESSY FACTOR	Moderate
PINTEREST TERMS	Kaleidoscope DIY simple, kaleidoscope craft for kids, paper towel roll kaleidoscope
GRADE LEVEL	Elementary and middle schools

essing the Group: Tip Sheet

troduction and Warm-Up Ideas

ve students view images of illusions to explore how different perspectives inform our thinking

ays to Grade or Modify the Activity

ve some purchased kaleidoscopes available to use and personalize them with stickers or words

e different materials to make the craft sturdier (e.g., polyvinyl chloride pipe)

uestions You May Want to Ask

ow have your personal values changed over time? What matters a lot to you now that you did not see as portant before?

ow have changes been challenging for you at school? What are some other perspectives that might provide u with a new way to see that change?

hat changes have actually led to outcomes that you now see as favorable?

hat skills are important when having to work through unexpected changes?

hat activities have you participated in that have been helpful to you when working through personal anges? What activities help you see different perspectives?

ow might the habit of trying to see change from different perspectives before assuming the worst help you pe with change?

hat is the role of other people in helping to see different perspectives?

hat personal strengths and skills do you have that can help work through changes beyond your control?

acilitation Strategies

rovide examples of how using the kaleidoscope could actually be a tool to help develop habits around deliberately exploring and considering different perspectives

ormalize that change is difficult and ambivalence is common

onsider the different stages of change and use strategies accordingly

Facilitator's Notes

- What current changes are causing students distress at school

- What skills do they identify as helping with coping

- Supports that will be used to help foster habits

Group #17

Jorge Ochoa, OTR/L

GROUP TITLE	Get Into the Groove: Experimenting With Rhythm
ACTIVITY	Drumming (collective drumming)
PURPOSE	The purpose of this therapeutic activity is to engage students in an activity that helps them **get in the groove** when they feel like their rhythm is off at school. While drumming together, students examine their habits and routines and consider how different activities may help them **get back into the groove** at school. Students in the drum circle are encouraged to explore progressively more difficult beats to create a cohesive group rhythm/sound. Group members can make parallels between the experience of the drum circle with the skills and strategies necessary to **"get into the groove"** during the school day. Additionally, the participants discuss how having a routine may help to **stay in the groove** during the school day. This therapeutic group is designed for students who have recent occupational issues and positive screens for: • High levels of stress during the day • Lacking a satisfying routine at school, which causes increased stress • Personal interests that are no longer part of routine • Not being able to focus on what one is doing • Difficulty adapting and coping to school stressors • Trouble completing school assignments and meeting expectations

SESSION GOALS	1. Participate in a drumming circle. 2. Adapt to a progressively more difficult rhythm or beat. 3. Consider how the experiences of **getting into the groove** during the drumm circle may help **getting back into the groove at school**.
OCCUPATION AS MEANS AND ENDS	This therapeutic group uses drumming as a means to invite students to consider changing their habits and routines to **get back into the groove** at school.
DIRECTIONS	This activity provides an opportunity for a unique experience each round. The basi steps of creating a drum or percussion circle include: 1. Have members of the circle select a percussion instrument. Give them some tir to get familiar with the sounds and explore how to hold and play the instrume 2. Arrange the group in a circle—it is a drum circle! 3. Identify one person to start a steady beat for the group. It might be helpful to start with a slower beat. Encourage everyone to focus on the rhythm. 4. Have everyone go around and copy that beat. 5. Invite someone to alternate the tempo (make it faster or slower), alternate the volume, and/or add a few extra beats to the original sequence. 6. Invite several people to **"get into the groove"** together and have fun!
MATERIALS	• Empty 5-gallon buckets (turned upside down) with equal pair of drumsticks, djembes, or frame drums • Shakers (maracas, eggs, custom made, etc.) • Armless chairs
MESSY FACTOR	Low
PINTEREST TERMS	Bucket drumming for kids, easy maracas for kids, paper cup music crafts, DIY hand drum, drumming up some fun
GRADE LEVEL	Elementary and early middle schools (easily adapted for all grade levels)

essing the Group: Tip Sheet

troduction and Warm-Up Ideas

ve group members make easy percussion instruments to use in the circle (maracas, tambourines, rhythm
cks)
k an open question to prepare them for the activity: "What's the difference between noise and harmony?"
ve some fun trying a humming circle to a popular song
ntrast doing something mindfully from mindlessly

ays to Grade or Modify the Activity

ve visual prompts (lights, adapted music sheets) to help synchronize the rhythm
ap or tap the beat with hands or feet

uestions You May Want to Ask

ow did drumming and listening to the beat help you to participate in an activity mindfully?
escribe your drumming performance when you could anticipate the rhythm. What similarities exist for
ur performance when there is a routine you can follow at school?
That other activities do you do that help you to become mindful and **get into the groove**? Do you expect
at these activities could help you **get back into the groove**?
That will the school day look like when you **get back into the groove** at school?
That skills and strategies can you work on to help **stay in the groove** when things change unexpectedly at
hool? What tools? What people?
That kinds of things can you achieve at school if you improve your habits and routines?
veryone in the circle was working in unison to keep the rhythm. In what ways might doing activities with
her people help change the rhythm of school for the better? Make it easier to **get back into the groove** at
hool?

acilitation Strategies

ighlight the skills that students are using to **get into the groove** and stay on beat
ighlight parallels between their experience of the activity and what is happening at school

Facilitator's Notes

- How students describe feeling out of rhythm or not in sync with school

- Different activities and interests that support mindfulness

- Ways they interacted as a collective group to find the rhythm and **stay in the groove**

- Supports that may help to foster habits

Group #18

Andrea Thinnes, OTD, OTR/L, FNAP
and Anna Domina, OTD, OTR/L

GROUP TITLE	CANtradictions: The Game of Considering Both Things as True
ACTIVITY	Storytelling game
PURPOSE	The primary purpose for this storytelling game is to explore aspects of life that may not always seem to be logical. During this storytelling game, players turn over a paradox one by one and provide examples of how that may have played out in their life or in someone's close to them. Working through paradox is a strategy for highlighting creative thinking that may lead to identifying new possibilities and better ways to cope with the demands of school–life balance. The goal is to support reframing from a "both-and" mindset and explore new strategies.

The primary purpose for this storytelling game is to explore aspects of life that may not always seem to be logical. During this storytelling game, players turn over a paradox one by one and provide examples of how that may have played out in their life or in someone's close to them. Working through paradox is a strategy for highlighting creative thinking that may lead to identifying new possibilities and better ways to cope with the demands of school–life balance. The goal is to support reframing from a "both-and" mindset and explore new strategies.

Exploring dimensions of life that do not always follow surface logic is a helpful way to develop new mindsets and habits. Occupationally well students are able to make positive activity choices at school while circumventing thinking traps associated with dichotomous/all-or-nothing thinking.

The group may be helpful for students whose school participation is languishing and who experience:

- Feeling stuck knowing what to do at school
- Challenges working with peers and teachers who hold different views or opinions
- Difficulty compromising with peers and working in a group
- Feeling confused about future goals
- Outcomes to be unfair and outside of their personal control

	• Anxiety about uncertainty
	• Difficulty finding reasons to look forward to going to school
	• Participation challenges for activities that do not align exactly with personal interests
SESSION GOALS	1. Promote positive peer and social interactions through active listening, coopera with others, and clear communication.
	2. Make positive choices about life situations that may have two correct options.
	3. Reflect with the group on responsible decision making by analyzing choices related to situations with "both-and" mindset.
OCCUPATION AS MEANS AND ENDS	Use a storytelling game to encourage the adoption of a new both-and perspective and new habits to support school–life balance.
DIRECTIONS	This storytelling group begins by explaining the purpose of the session is to try and turn **con**tradictions in our lives into **can**tradictions by questioning the potential usefulness of different mindsets that accept two things at once rather than mindset that adopt more rigid ways of examining life events. The game starts with an exam of a paradox: The last born is the first to play—Get it? (The person is both last and f at the same time!) They turn over the first paradox card and read it aloud and start the 2-minute timer. Each player tries to come up with the best example for how the paradox applies to school. A rotating judge (or the therapist) decides which exampl most clearly upholds the paradox at school and awards the point each round. The player with the most points wins bragging rights and concludes the game with this paradoxical quote: **"Losing is just as much a part of a game as winning. They a equals."**
MATERIALS	• Paradox cards (the therapist is encouraged to add to the few provided)
	• Timer
	• Scorecard or tokens (optional)
MESSY FACTOR	Low
PINTEREST TERMS	Friends of irony, ironic jokes, paradox pictures
GRADE LEVEL	High school

Unwillingness to experience failure might mean that you may usually feel like you are failing.	Sleep is great for your health but doing it in school is only great for detention.
It is common to chase happiness and just as common to not do the things we know make us happy.	It is usually only when we accept our imperfections that we can even begin to work on changing them.
Social media brings a lot of people together and is equally responsible for disconnecting others.	Power can just as easily help one rise as it can make one fall.
We are social beings and solitude is one of the best ways to make one more sociable.	The only constant in life is usually change.

The thing that is usually most certain is uncertainty.	It's common to want to have choices, and too many choices can make it impossible to ever decide.
The best way to learn most things is through failure.	The more that one knows, the more one realizes all that they do not know.
The best way to sometimes say more is to talk less.	When we try too hard to keep something close, we usually end up pushing it farther away.

Thinking in Gray
(how I have worked through this paradox before …)

(Alternative way to play card)

essing the Group: Tip Sheet

troduction and Warm-Up Ideas

ve the group read some age- and school-appropriate jokes about ironic/paradoxical parts of life
view some funny paradoxical memes
actice naming upsides and downsides or pros and cons of certain topics
scuss the differences between a "both-and" and "either-or" mindset

ays to Grade or Modify the Activity

velop scenarios that are school-based that explore different paradoxes if it is too difficult for them to come
with their own examples
k students to come up with the solution to the two contradictory situations being true at the same time vs.
example of how that may have been relevant in their lives

uestions You May Want to Ask

ow do two competing values challenge the way you approach school or your current school–life balance?
hen you become unstuck, what activities do you imagine will be easier to incorporate into your daily rou-
ne? How might these activities help reinforce a both-and mindset?
hat two contradictory things may be true right now that are impacting your school performance in ways
at are not personally satisfying?
hat aspects of the school environment seem to be contradictory? How might you be able to use your ability
recognize possibilities to offer a solution?
hat outcomes do you imagine for yourself when your school–life balance improves?
hat do you imagine is the next best action for you to take?

acilitation Strategies

ormalize that change is usually preceded by feeling stuck
onsider using visuals to reinforce the two contradictory experiences and the alternative possibilities
elp to brainstorm alternative possibilities and possible plans for making changes

Facilitator's Notes

- Issues for which the students are experiencing ambivalence or feeling stuck

- Change talk (what they think they can do, want to do, need to do, have done before)

- Ways that possibilities were offered

- Next steps for making the change(s)

Group #19

*Paula Cook, OTD, OTR/L
and Ashley Fecht, OTD, OTR/L, BCP*

GROUP TITLE	Helping Myself By Helping Others: Toiletry Drive Care Packages
ACTIVITY	Toiletry drive
PURPOSE	The primary purpose for this school-wide toiletry drive is to promote empathy, responsibility for personal behaviors, and opportunities to repair one's reputation for actions that have caused harm or disrespect to others at school. The project enables students to be assigned to important roles and responsibilities to foster an occupational identity based on wanting to be more accepting and considerate of other people. Moreover, a toiletry drive provides students with practice helping others and may enable personal reflection that supports changing habits that were previously hurtful to others. The group may be helpful for students whose attitude at school has become progressively more negative and may present with occupational challenges, including: <ul><li>Putting others down and displaying a disrespectful attitude toward others</li><li>Lacking inhibition and dismissing school/classroom rules</li><li>Participating in vandalism of school property</li><li>Having difficulty relating to peers and forming friendships</li><li>Using aggressive behaviors to manipulate others perceived as weaker</li><li>Getting in trouble for fighting/bullying others at school</li></ul>

SESSION GOALS	1. Organize a toiletry drive at school. 2. Determine different tasks needed to complete the event. 3. Assign responsibilities and roles to group members. 4. Design a process for announcing details to other members of the school and community. 5. Explore organizations that would benefit from the donations. (It may take several sessions to develop a full plan.)
OCCUPATION AS MEANS AND ENDS	This Tier 2 group uses the occupation of organizing and participating in a toiletry donation drive to facilitate opportunities to fulfill roles and take responsibility for making a positive contribution to the school-wide community.
DIRECTIONS	This group activity has three distinct phases: planning and informing the school of toiletry drive, building toiletry kits for chosen organizations or causes, and donating the completed kits. The first phase focuses on identifying a community organization inquiring after their most-desired toiletry items, establishing a timeline, and creating a daily schedule for handling the incoming inventory and responsibilities. The second phase likely requires creating a message about the drive, setting up bins, collecting items that were donated, and sorting supplies into kits. The last phase involves transferring the kits to the organization in need.
MATERIALS	• Flyers/advertisements • A drop-off bin • A variety of toiletries • Quart-size zipper bags • Personalized notes for each bag
MESSY FACTOR	Low
PINTEREST TERMS	Blessing bag checklist, homeless kits, random acts of kindness, comfort bags, free printable notes
GRADE LEVEL	Middle and high schools

[NAME OF SCHOOL]
IS EXCITED TO HOST A
TOILETRY DRIVE

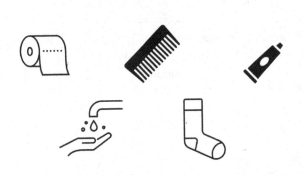

[INSERT DATES]

ms Needed to Help the Community

eodorant	Sunscreen	Socks
and sanitizer	Sanitary supplies	Soap
oothbrush	Combs	Diapers
oothpaste	Shampoo	Conditioner
Mouthwash	Lotion	Shaving cream
isposable razors	Toilet paper	Lip balm

ease drop off your donations in the (insert location; e.g., big blue bins) on campus between (insert dates). our donations help (list the organization[s] that will receive the kits and their respective causes).

anks for making a difference!

Example Bin Flyer

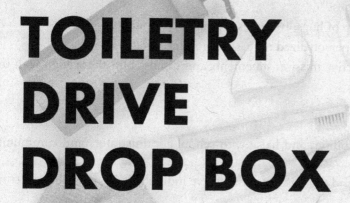

TOILETRY
DRIVE
DROP BOX

Unused and unopened!

Don't have anything?

Go get some to benefit _____! ☺

Due:

essing the Group: Tip Sheet

troduction and Warm-Up Ideas

ive the group brainstorm a recipe for "kindness"

ve them some support if needed (e.g., ½ cup of hugs, 10 smiles, a pinch of hospitality)

u can use this group-developed recipe as a personalized note to put in each toiletry kit

search local organizations and their respective mission statements and discuss how these align with the
oup's values and kits

ays to Grade or Modify the Activity

ssume some of the organizational responsibilities and liaise with school administrators and community
cial service organizations

ovide students with a list of area agencies and organizations that serve individuals who may benefit from
care package

uestions You May Want to Ask

ow does becoming recognized as a caring person fit with your personal values?

ow does practicing caring for others and doing selfless activities support you in being able to care for your-
lf and see your personal qualities in a different light?

hat kinds of activities can support you in developing a habit around giving back and caring for others?
ow will this lend itself to a more positive reputation among others in the school community?

ow have your behaviors with others caused challenges for you at school? How have consequences inhibited
u from being able to participate in things that matter to you?

hat changes do you feel are necessary for becoming more known as someone who cares about others and
chool? How willing are you to make those changes?

Meeting obligations and handling responsibilities is a way to feel competent about ourselves. What skills did
u use for completing tasks for this toiletry drive?

hat outcomes do you imagine for yourself the next time you are given responsibilities for projects at school?

acilitation Strategies

upport students in articulating how participation in the activities is helping them

Make a list and revisit it often

upport self-efficacy by identifying and sharing your observations of skills they are using well as they work
n different parts of the project

Help to manage the daily task list so that you can monitor how students handle responsibilities

Help to create a checklist of all the tasks that will be needed to fully complete the project

rovide positive feedback when tasks are completed well

Facilitator's Notes

- What the students reported in terms of skills

- How occupational engagement supported improved participation in other valued roles

- Changes and expectations for success in making the change

- Values clarification to support desired occupational identity (e.g., "I'm a caring person")

Group #20

Marcela De La Pava, MS, OTR/L
and Laurette Olson, PhD, OTR/L, FAOTA

GROUP TITLE	Sending the Rocket to Inner Space
ACTIVITY	Craft

PURPOSE	The primary purpose for this craft activity is to support children in learning how to use their breath as a tool for self-regulation. The students make a straw rocket toy and then are supported in using it as a tool to explore **inner** space. Additionally, the occupational therapy practitioner explores how the rocket can be used throughout the school day to help them practice deep breathing. Students discuss how being able to better manage their emotions and behaviors will support them in being able to better complete school tasks and responsibilities.
	Self-regulation is a key skill that is needed for children to succeed in classroom group activities. They must be able to regulate their physical and emotional states so they can control their impulses and behavior to support their group participation and to develop and maintain good relationships with teachers and classmates.

	The group may be helpful for students who are languishing emotionally and experience the following occupational concerns: • Exhibit emotional outbursts in class that cause disruptions to self and other learn • Have difficulty relating to peers and forming friendships • Feel overwhelmed by school tasks • Feel large amount of stress at school • Break school or classroom rules • Have difficulty coping with and adapting to changes at school
SESSION GOALS	1. Complete the rocket craft. 2. Send the **rocket to inner space** by practicing deep breathing. 3. Identify a schedule for sending the **rocket to inner space** during the school da
OCCUPATION AS MEANS AND ENDS	Using a craft activity to build habits around self-regulation and encourage activity choices that better meet the expectations of the student role.
DIRECTIONS	This activity provides students with an opportunity to complete a quick straw rocke craft. Students are provided with instructions, visuals to help with sizing, and safety strategies for cutting and hot gluing. The craft takes about 10 minutes to complete and uses common supplies. The main focus of the activity is to brainstorm how the rocket toy can be used at different times during the school day to help them manag their emotions and better meet classroom rules and more fully participate in the student role.
MATERIALS	• Standard straws • Smoothie or milkshake straws • Duct tape • Craft cardboard or colored foam • Hot glue gun • Scissors
MESSY FACTOR	Medium
PINTEREST TERMS	Space rocket straw craft, straw rocket, printable straw rockets, balloon rocket, frugal fun, DIY straw blowers
GRADE LEVEL	Preschool and early elementary school

v Rocket Instructions

Cut a strip of the milkshake/wider straw the length of the line below:

_____

Seal one end of the straw with duct tape. You want to make sure that no air can escape.

Make the rocket fins by cutting three small triangles out of foam or cardboard. If you need a stencil, you can use the triangle below:

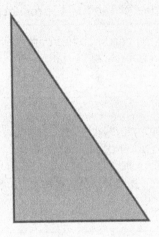

. Now glue your fins to the base of the straw. Before you glue them, you may want to decorate the fins with designs or words that will encourage you to take deep breaths.

. Load the rocket onto the smaller straw. Take a deep breath. Blow. Now feel the difference in your inner space after taking a big, long breath!

Calming Scale

After sending my rocket to outer space, my inner space felt:

(Try to do it until you feel like the smiling face.)

essing the Group: Tip Sheet

troduction and Warm-Up Ideas

t up a straw race and have them count the number of times they had to blow until the cotton ball crossed
e finish line; have them compare their numbers

sure the finish line is far enough away to encourage several breaths

ays to Grade or Modify the Activity

ve students make a few rockets (one for school, one for home, one for out in the community)

ve students strategize how they are going to store and keep up with the toy at school so it does not get
maged and they can access it when they need to take deep breaths

uestions You May Want to Ask

ow does taking care of your **inner space** (i.e., body, mind, breath) help you to do the things you need to do
school?

ow might you have more success by using the tool to help you stay feeling good and positive rather than
aiting until you do not feel good?

hat are some of the strategies that are the same for helping us take care of ourselves and helping us take care
our belongings and toys, like this new rocket?

hat kinds of things can you achieve at school if you get better at being able to keep yourself calm and do
ur deep breathing exercises?

ow might being more calm help you be the best friend you can be?

ow might being more calm help you better perform your favorite activities at school?

hat would it look like if you developed a habit of breathing several times a day at school?

acilitation Strategies

rovide examples of how using the toy could be used at different times during the school day

elp them to understand the importance of using the toy *before* they feel upset or overwhelmed

Facilitator's Notes

- What students noted were their favorite activities

- How the toy supports self-regulation habits

- Ways that using it to prevent feeling overwhelmed and upset were discussed

- Supports that will be used to help foster habits

Group #21

Ashley Stoffel, OTD, OTR/L, FAOTA
and Jane Clifford O'Brien, PhD, OTR/L, FAOTA

GROUP TITLE	Hooping for Hope
ACTIVITY	Hula hooping, jumping, hopscotch
PURPOSE	The purpose of this therapeutic group is to encourage students to explore and discover how hope can be fostered through different activities. Specifically, the group activities consist of traditional hula hooping, as well as using the hula hoop as a proxy for a jump rope and using the hoops to create a hopscotch pattern. The goal is to help them look at how they manage the challenges presented in the hula hooping activities as a way to explore the possibility of overcoming current obstacles or challenges that might be contributing to their negative attitude at school. Students are encouraged to consider how the strategies used to hoop well in each activity might apply to how they can approach different challenges at school. Using everyday activities that reinforce skilled performance can help to facilitate a sense of capacity. Students who feel more capable and skillful are more likely to expect success, persist in school activities that are challenging, and cope adaptively to changes. Facilitators encourage **thinking more hopefully** about successful school outcomes by reinforcing how group members persisted, used objects in new or novel ways, and worked hard to get their proper footing.

	The group may be helpful for students who are experiencing occupational issues a school and present more recently as: • Being highly self-critical and having an inaccurate sense of abilities • Withdrawing owing to fear of failure • Having a sense of impending doom; **feeling hopeless** • Having increased feelings of anxiety • Doubting abilities to complete school tasks • Lacking confidence about self as a student, friend, or peer • Focusing only on the negative aspects of school experiences
SESSION GOALS	1. Complete the activities using hula hoops. 2. Make a list of skills that were used to overcome challenges in the activities and perform them competently.
OCCUPATION AS MEANS AND ENDS	Use hula hooping activities to support students in more accurately appraising their abilities and strengthening their occupational identities as students, friends, and pee
DIRECTIONS	This group is made up of a series of different physical activities that can be done wi a hula hoop: traditional hula hooping around the waist and some tricks, jumping wi a hula hoop instead of a jump rope, and completing a hopscotch pattern created from different hula hoops. In each activity, students are asked to examine their performance. While engaging in traditional hula hooping fun, students are prompte to think about how often they got right back into the activity after the hoop fell, ho they naturally picked the hoop back up, and how they moved themselves to try and keep the hoop from falling. They may also be encouraged to try to flow with multip hoops at the same time and discuss how they kept several things from falling down once. They may also be supported in trying to hoop with different parts of the body (e.g., arm, elbow, leg). In the second activity, students consider how they recovered after being tripped up and what it was like to jump through hoops. In the final hopscotch activity, students are invited to consider the strategies needed for keepin their footing to match the hopscotch pattern.
MATERIALS	• Several different sized hula hoops (preferably two small and one large diameter for each participant)
MESSY FACTOR	Low
PINTEREST TERMS	Hula hoop outdoor play, hula hoop showdown, fun hula hoop games, hula hoop beginner tricks
GRADE LEVEL	Elementary school

essing the Group: Tip Sheet

troduction and Warm-Up Ideas

l them to line up holding hands

ce a hula hoop over the first person's free arm and have them work together to move the hoop down the
e

t up a ring toss target and have each participant name a worry they are going to try and toss out of their
nd during the group

ays to Grade or Modify the Activity

ake this a three-series group and focus each group on one of the activities

emonstrate hula hooping with hands and arms if waist is too difficult to encourage a successful experience

erapist also hoops to show they experience challenges too

uestions You May Want to Ask

rt of being successful at hooping is picking it up as soon as it falls and starting again. What might be going
i in your life right now that could benefit from that same strategy? What matters enough to you to try a
w approach?

hat personal strengths and characteristics help you to stay engaged with activities that might be challeng-
g or require you to start over?

mping with the hula hoop has a lot to do with timing the jump just right. Are there any goals you have that
ay just need a little more time before you get it just right? What do you think it will be like when you finally
hieve that goal?

hen the hoop starts spinning out of control, we can adjust our position to get better control. What are some
rengths you have used in the past to help you get better control of some things that seemed to be spinning
it of control? How did that experience increase your sense of hope?

opscotch requires us to think about our footing. Life can sometimes throw our footing off and make us feel
elpless or hopeless. What strategies did you use to help you keep your footing? How does being grounded
nd having good footing prepare you to be more successful? More hopeful?

his activity had you jumping through hoops. What kinds of things are going on in your life that might leave
ou feeling like you have had to jump through hoops? What strategies have we discussed that might help
nake the situation seem more hopeful? What strengths do you have that might help?

acilitation Strategies

how children new ways to do things and move with the hula hoop in fun ways before they show signs of
rustration or boredom

eep activities fun and noncompetitive

oint out children's strengths

Facilitator's Notes

- Things that students indicated mattered to them

- How occupation encouraged reflecting on skills to build volition and a stronger occupational identity

- How the therapist modeled persistence responding to challenges

Group #22

Jessica Weiler, OTD, OTR/L, CTRP
and Megan Eads, BSHS, OTD, OTR/L

GROUP TITLE	Thyme to Relax
ACTIVITY	Gardening (container)
PURPOSE	This therapeutic group begins with creating a classroom-based herb garden and a rotation of responsibilities to support students in practicing embedding restorative and nonacademic tasks into their daily routine at school. The goal is to support students who are at risk for academic burnout and who need support to intentionally set aside time to relax and recharge. Gardening activities were chosen because they provide students with caretaking tasks that can be done mindfully and support them in developing the habit of taking a break for mental well-being during the school day. Strategies to increase their commitment for restorative occupations to help overall skill and performance are discussed. Additionally, students self-monitor their state of relaxation before and after the activity and are encouraged to commit to this habit. Occupationally well students are able to identify and routinely participate in calming and relaxing activities at school to effectively cope with stress and decrease levels of anxiety. Occupationally well students have daily routines that include restorative occupations. The group may be helpful for students who are languishing emotionally and who may lack occupational strategies to: • Decrease the risk of school burnout or exhaustion • Intentionally engage in restorative occupations • Avoid the unhealthy traps of perfectionism • Avoid overcommitting self to clubs and extracurricular activities • Decrease the risk for dropping out of school • Adopt a healthier balance between rest and productivity

	• Implement rest and sleep routines needed to adequately complete tasks • Work through feelings of being overwhelmed by the pressures of school • Develop an accurate perspective on failure and performance capacity (there a[r] not unending reservoirs of energy and mental endurance)

SESSION GOALS	1. Start a small classroom container herb garden.
	2. Practice mindful gardening strategies while planting herbs.
	3. Make a list of daily tasks needed to care for plants.
	4. Create a daily garden schedule and assign participants.
	5. Have students commit to gardening mindfully and recording their pre-/post-st[r]
	   levels.
	6. Identify parallels between the care needed to keep the garden alive and thrivi[ng]
	   and the care needed to keep oneself mentally well and thriving at school.

OCCUPATION AS MEANS AND ENDS	School gardening is used to promote building a routine that includes restorative occupation and habits that promote mindfulness and relaxation.
DIRECTIONS	Group members are asked to create a classroom herb garden from seeds. Whether you have an existing school garden, are trying to create one, or are working within a confined space, gardening can be done on any scale and is incredibly beneficial for students to be part of the process. This group activity uses a small-scale garden design. Students need to investigate the recommended care for each plant and wri[te] it on the stake. They plant the seeds and develop a rotating restorative schedule for attending to gardening tasks and caring for the herbs. Participants are given a variet[y] of materials, including various pictures of small-scale herb gardens but no exact instructions on how their garden should look. They commit to trying not to think about anything but caring for the plants as a wa[y] to offer themselves needed respite from the pressures of school. In addition, they us[e] the garden occupation as a way to apply and practice mindfulness skills in the conte[xt] of an occupation. Before and after the activity, students report their overall mood an[d] relaxation level to help build self-monitoring strategies and more effectively see the impact of restorative occupations on supporting relaxation. They also use the pulse oximeter to measure biometric information before and after and are encouraged to stay engaged until stress levels have fallen (oxygen saturation levels are 95% or high[er])
MATERIALS	• Containers for individual herb plants • Seeds • Potting soil or dirt • Watering pail • Garden stakes • Pruning shears • Schedule template • Small cartons or containers, paper towel rolls

	• Gardening trowel • Leaves • Grass • Sticks • Wood bark • Sand • Small to medium rocks • Small toys, such as dolls, LEGO pieces, dinosaurs, or cars • Small plants • Gardening gloves • Cleaning materials: soap, water, wipes/towels • Fertilizer • Glue, tape • Whimsical craft supplies (glitter, colored feathers, poms) • Clothespins • Popsicle sticks • Pulse oximeter
ESSY CTOR	High for getting garden set up; low for routine maintenance and harvesting of the herbs
NTEREST RMS	School garden, meditation garden, calming garden, zen garden, restorative garden, whimsical garden, magical garden, fairy garden for kids, sensory garden, herb garden, indoor herbs, community garden, herbs, farm stand, plants and mood, restorative plants, oxygen and plants
RADE VEL	Middle and high schools

cessing the Group: Tip Sheet

ntroduction and Warm-Up Ideas

Review simple herb-based recipes (e.g., olive oil and dried herb dipping sauce, herb-infused soaps)

Practice a relaxation and mood report together

Explore different mobile mood and relaxation trackers

Practice using the pulse oximeter and doing deep breathing to see its impact on biometric data

Ways to Grade or Modify the Activity

Eliminate the biometric readings

Making mindfulness cue cards or posters in the garden area to encourage integrating these strategies during the task

Consider how often the group should reconvene to discuss progress

Questions You May Want to Ask

- What parts of the school day do you imagine would be the easiest times for you to incorporate rest activities into your routine?
- How does stress impact your performance at school? During other activities that are personally mea to you?
- What aspects of your academic performance do you value the most? How might these factors be en by restoring yourself and energy?
- What strategies have you used in the past to develop healthy habits for yourself? Which of those m helpful to you in building a healthy routine around rest?
- What changes do you think may be possible?

Facilitation Strategies

- Make sure to reinforce that developing habits is the priority and not the quality of the garden and har
- Help them to identify a robust list of tasks so they stay engaged sufficiently in the restorative occupati
- Provide instructions on how to ensure the experience is truly restorative and not a chore (do ever mindfully, focus on being with the plants and caring for them vs. doing garden chores)

Daily Mood and Relaxation Mental Health Log

Overall, I would rate my mood at school today as (place an "X"):

Awful	Not So Good	Just Okay	Pretty Good	Amazing

If you selected awful or not so good, have you reached out to anyone you trust or used any of your mental promotion strategies?

Overall, I would rate my level of relaxation at school right now as (place an "X"):

Very Relaxed						Very Stresse

What did the pulse oximeter report before starting the activity? Consider including your biometric data be

ardening activities do you intend to do today? Remember to do them mindfully. Spend time being with the nd keeping your promise of trying to clear your mind, and get some energy back to finish the rest of the to be with the garden for at least 10 minutes.

Tasks for Today	Mindfulness or Relaxation Strategy

, after the activity, I would rate my mood at school right now as (place an "X"):

Awful	Not So Good	Just Okay	Pretty Good	Amazing

, after the activity, I would rate my level of relaxation at school right now as (place an "X"):

Very Relaxed					Very Stressed

did the pulse oximeter report after gardening? Consider including your biometric data below.

Facilitator's Notes

- How data tracking can help with habit development

- Change-management strategies for aspects of change they anticipate will be successful

- Anticipated impact of restoration on academic performance

- Doing occupation mindfully

Group #23

Ingris Treminio, DrOT, OT/L, BCP

GROUP TITLE	Making the Media Social: No More Waiting in the Wings
ACTIVITY	Art mural and photography
PURPOSE	This therapeutic group focuses on cultivating a sense of belonging for students who may not be participating fully in school activities. The small group intervention helps students to plan a selfie challenge at school and engage in a collaborative mural project. The goal of the installation is to encourage students to **stop waiting in the wings** and to **start spreading their wings** by creating a large wing mural space for everyone to celebrate themselves and encourage a collective sense of belonging. As students engage in creating the wing mural, the occupational therapy facilitator asks them to explore how habits of isolating, withdrawing, self-imposing activity restrictions, and limiting social interactions may be setting them up to **wait in the wings** rather than learning how to **spread their wings**. They explore how contributing to the social fabric of school may align with future goals or aspirations and help to develop valued friendships and relationships. The total experience is expected to support students in making a connection between participating in occupations and opportunities to show pride, becoming more visible within the community, and reflecting on their individual contributions to the greater school community.

Occupationally well students report positive relationships and positive experiences interacting with peers at school. Students who feel they are accepted and have a strong sense of belonging at school have better academic outcomes and greater mental well-being.

The group may be helpful for students who are presenting with the following occupational concerns:

- Withdrawing socially from classmates and interactions at school
- Limiting participation because they wonder if they have anything to contribute to the school community
- Isolating because they do not expect others to enjoy their company or want to be friends with them
- Engaging in mostly solitary activities owing to feeling different or worrying they will be judged or bullied for being different

	• Not feeling worthy or good enough to be liked by other peers • Unhealthy self-concept and not feeling pride in their skills or what they accomplish • Reporting a minimal or restricted sense of belonging at school
SESSION GOALS	1. Discuss how small group activities and occupation can cultivate opportunities strengthen one's sense of belonging at school. 2. Decide which wing mural to do after independently reviewing options. 3. Design the mural. 4. Invite the school to participate. (It is likely this small group intervention will require several sessions to fully organize the project from start to finish.)
OCCUPATION AS MEANS AND ENDS	This group uses an art mural and photography to promote engagement with other students while focusing on developing a sense of belonging by shifting performance patterns from **waiting in the wings** to **spreading their wings** at school.
DIRECTIONS	In this therapeutic group, the media becomes social! Students are instructed to create an interactive mural either in the classroom (bulletin board) or within the larger school environment. The theme for the larger interactive mural is **no more waiting in the wings** as a way to encourage social participation and to celebrate each student's unique contribution to the greater school community. The student group decides what kind of wings they will make (e.g., angel, butterfly, airplane) and begins constructing a large right and left wing. Each student contributes to constructing the mural, discussing the caption or hashtag, and inviting students in the school to the selfie challenge. They are also responsible for developing a plan to see if the space they created in the school brought people together. The facilitator offers guidance throughout the project.
MATERIALS	• Large roll of paper to create the outline of the wings • Big cardboard boxes or poster boards • A variety of arts and craft supplies (Washi tape, easy-peel tapes, markers, paint supplies, chalk) • Glue • Command hooks to position and hold each wing • Paper to make flyers and invitations to announce the selfie challenge • A step stool or ladder to hang the mural (Students have to problem solve the design based on supplies available.)
MESSY FACTOR	High
PINTEREST TERMS	Kids feather wings mural, interactive street art, selfie wall ideas
GRADE LEVEL	Elementary, middle, and high schools

essing the Group: Tip Sheet

troduction and Warm-Up Ideas

view different memes about self-worth
ok at different interactive wings murals

ays to Grade or Modify the Activity

esign the group to span multiple sessions
e the dry-erase board for the selfie wall
eate a team who will change out the mural periodically
e the mural to give extra attention to social issues that are important in the school community

uestions You May Want to Ask

what ways did the group activity allow you to consider how engaging in activities with others can help you become a more visible member of the school community?
hat activities may help you to develop or strengthen valued friendships?
ow do you imagine the selfie wall or interactive mural will create a greater sense of community at school?
hat skills did you contribute to this project? How might you contribute those skills in other ways at school?
what ways might some of your social habits be interfering with making meaningful relationships with ers at school?
hat changes do you anticipate for yourself the next time you have the choice to do things socially with ers? How will you use this experience to commit to **not waiting in the wings**?

acilitation Strategies

rovide guidance, particularly for scale with respect to time and available supplies
eek potential collaborators, like the art teacher, maintenance staff, or drama teacher
elp with designing the process for inviting members of the school to take the selfie challenge and how to mply collect data on who uses the wall
iscuss strategies for rotating the installation
ffer this as an after-school group or extracurricular activity

Facilitator's Notes

- Interactions that supported group cohesion

- Ways the occupation supported showing pride/being excited for the school to use the space

- Individual's contributions to the greater process and project/how each person contributed to something
er than themselves

ol Selfie Challenge Announcement

'/e are inviting everyone (including teachers and staff) to participate in the school
elfie challenge from _____ to _____ [dates]. The mural was created
y fellow students. We hope you enjoy!

Add a hashtag to your photo to honor something positive you do at school:

Doing something you are good at

Talking with someone you admire or care about

Taking care of the school grounds or property

Sharing something with a peer

Feeling proud

Teaching someone a new activity you enjoy

Helping someone

Cleaning up something

Showing school spirit

Being a role model

Being authentically you!

Mural Examples

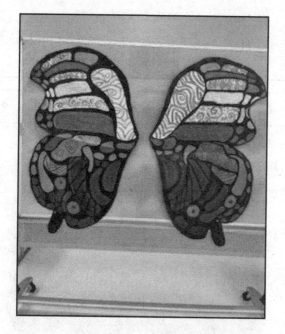
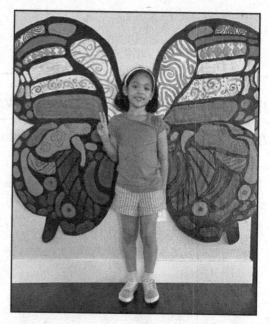
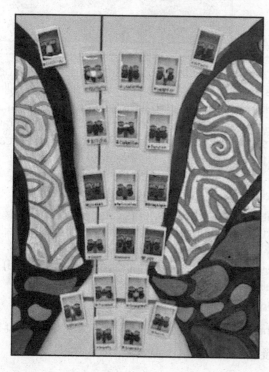
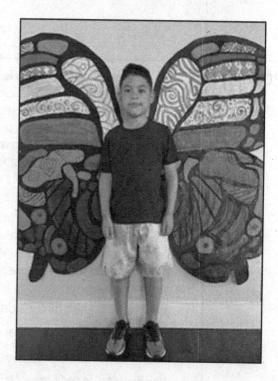

Group #24

*Kelsey Helgesen, OTR/L
and Brad E. Egan, OTD, PhD, CADC, OTR/L*

OUP TITLE	Be(ad) in the Moment: Coping With Grief and Loss
TIVITY	Jewelry (bracelet) making and storytelling

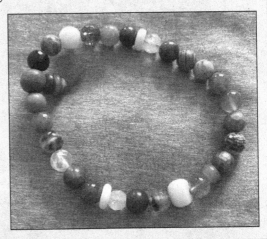

RPOSE	The purpose of this Tier 2 group is to support students who are struggling at school after a recent personal loss. Students engage in an activity that combines storytelling and jewelry making to promote healing. The occupational therapy professional also explores how students can incorporate the bracelet into a daily ritual of remembrance when grief seems overwhelming at school, especially because effective routines can be helpful for coping with grief and loss. Students also identify how occupations and meaningful activities support working through grief and loss, are effective in preserving important memories, and encourage **be(ad)ing in the moment**.

The healing bracelet story is occupation-focused so students can memorialize an important relationship in the context of how it impacted themselves occupationally. The personal story can be read daily in conjunction with touching or moving the beads on the bracelet to create a new ritual and devote intentional time to **be(ad) in the moment** and work through feelings of grief and loss at school.

The group may be helpful for students with occupational concerns who are:

- Unable to or struggle to meet the expectations of student role after significant loss

- Feeling overwhelmed by grief at school

- Withdrawing socially from classmates and interactions at school

- Experiencing behavioral changes that are interfering with following classroom and school rules, turning things in on time, and/or school attendance

- Unable to concentrate or keep their mind on school tasks and responsibilities

SESSION GOALS	1. Complete the therapeutic story and accompanying bracelet. 2. Discuss how grief and loss impact school participation. 3. Explore how to strengthen performance patterns to mitigate some of the scho challenges caused by recent grief and loss.
OCCUPATION AS MEANS AND ENDS	This therapeutic group uses jewelry making and storytelling to support healing an strengthen performance patterns to meet school expectations while addressing personal grief and loss.
DIRECTIONS	Students are given a fill-in-the-blank story that attempts to memorialize an importa relationship. Each blank relates back to important occupational information that ma be helpful for using occupation to work through grief and loss. After the student completes the story, they begin to construct the healing bracelet according to the details and suggested order of the beads written into the story. If a student needs more beads added to the bracelet owing to wrist size, clear beads are added to preserve the story's color scheme. Once the bracelet is completed, the group pract using the story and bracelet's beads to complete a quick memory meditation by touching each bead as the story is read in full. Thoughts on incorporating this new ritual into one's everyday life are discussed, along with the value of everyday routine on working through the grief cycle.
MATERIALS	• A wide assortment of jewelry beads • Elastic bracelet string • Scissors • A customized story (facilitator may have to make some adjustments to the story based on age and reading level, available supplies, etc.)
MESSY FACTOR	Low
PINTEREST TERMS	Healing bracelet, in memory of loss jewelry, story bracelet kids, beaded bracelet idea
GRADE LEVEL	All grade levels

...nories That Help Me Get Through the Day: A Bracelet Story of You and Me

_____

...k of you often. What I remember most about you is _____ **(insert dark red stone)**. Sometimes I
...ad. That's just a part of this. Thinking of you also makes me happy. When I need to smile, I can always
... of these three things about you: _____, _____ and _____ **(insert three blue stones)**.
...n I need a good laugh, I just remember the time that you and I _____ **(insert green stone)**.

...gnize parts of you in me. That also makes me happy. One of the values I get from you is _____
...**rt wooden stone)**. When I do well at something, I can imagine you thinking _____ **(insert orange
...e)**. Thank you for being positive in those moments. There are many different skills I learned from you.
...skills, in particular, I am pretty proud of are _____ and _____ **(insert two silver stones)**. Thank
...or helping me practice those skills.

...if I may be sad at times, the memories I have of you help me keep going. One of my favorite things
...o is still _____ **(insert light blue stone)**. I also think about different places we went together. One
...e that I always associate you with is _____ **(insert multicolor stone)**. When I feel overwhelmed by
...I can go to _____ **(insert brown stone)**. I can actually think about you wherever I go!

...y things about my day have changed, but I try to make sure I still do _____ **(insert pink stone)**
...y day. That was something you reminded me was important. Another part of my routine that you'd
...appy has not changed is _____ **(insert red stone)**. It helps me get through the day just like the
...nories I have of you do.

...so thankful for the memories. They help each day seem better. I carry you in my heart. I know you carry
...oo. This final bead of the bracelet story **(insert bead of your choice)** represents something I hope you
...ys remember about me: _____.

...nk you for the memories. Thank you for this story I can read when I want to think about you. Thank you
...for this new bracelet, which gives me another way to carry around our memories.

...n: _____

Consider making your own beads out of paper! Students could write messages or memories on the paper strips as another way to memorialize someone important to them.

Paper Bead Instructions

1. Cut strips of paper about ½ inch wide and about 12 inches long.

2. Decorate the paper by adding designs, color, and messages. It is also possible to use paper strips ma from wrapping, scrapbook, and/or craft paper.

3. Use a small dowel or skewer to roll the paper up tightly.

4. Add a small dab of glue to the small end and smooth out with your fingers.

5. Gently remove the bead from the dowl. Consider painting the bead with glitter nail polish or a craft to help it harden and shine.

6. Let them dry completely and string them on your bracelet!

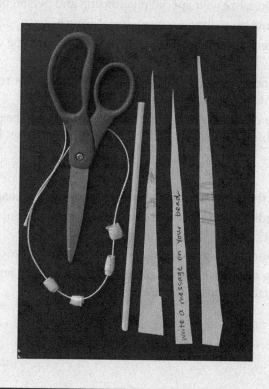

essing the Group: Tip Sheet

troduction and Warm-Up Ideas

scuss the normal experiences of grief after a significant loss

ve a moment of silence to honor all the special people and relationships the students are grieving

eate a grief and loss occupational checklist and see how many each person identifies with

ays to Grade or Modify the Activity

ovide students with a story customized to grade and literacy level

onsider having the activity span a few group sessions

eate a necklace, keychain, or other personal accessory

uestions You May Want to Ask

what ways did the group activity allow you to be present in your grief process?

hat activities help you memorialize your special relationship and person best?

hat features of the school environment (places or people) have been supportive of your grief process?

re there ways you have figured out to successfully grieve at school or cope with feelings as they might arise nexpectedly?

ow might certain activities help you cope with grief in ways that do not result in more pain and suffering actions that are inconsistent with your typical school behavior?

hat kind of changes do you expect to see in your daily routine as you begin to cope more adaptively and turn to doing some of the things you did regularly before your significant loss?

acilitation Strategies

ormalize grief and loss and the occupational changes that may be expected

onsider having a closing meditation activity that allows them to be present with their grief and practice us- g the story and bracelet as a ritual

ave some extra supplies so one can easily exchange beads based on the size of the student's wrist and bracelet

iscuss strategies for building memorializing rituals and routines and the potential of stable daily routines to ring a sense of wellness or stability during the grief process

Facilitator's Notes

- Successful adaptive strategies of using occupations and activities to be present with grief and work th[rough] difficult and unexpected emotions

- Ways that occupations were discussed to offer a way to memorialize important relationships

- The role of routines and rituals in working through grief and loss

Group #25

Teri K. Rupp, MOT, OTR/L, C/NDT
and Patricia Bowyer, EdD, MS, OTR, FAOTA, SFHEA

OUP TITLE	Eyes Off the Road—HELP!
TIVITY	Racing remote control cars
RPOSE	This small group intervention addresses self-efficacy and supports students in exploring how feedback from others can be helpful to understanding one's own abilities and effectiveness. Students in the group have to use feedback from other members to successfully steer remote control cars while blindfolded. They will surely need the help of others because their **eyes are off the road**. The occupational therapy facilitator assists students in identifying parallels between this group activity and situations that occur at school when their **eyes may be off the road** and they stand to benefit from objective feedback from others. In particular, students explore how objective feedback might be a way to help them **keep their eyes on the road at school** and avoid some of the challenges that may occur owing to thinking traps like accepting helplessness, judging oneself unfairly, and perfectionism. Occupationally well students have a good sense of their own abilities and efficacy. They are able to effectively make activity choices or develop strategies to improve skills needed for school tasks. They understand the importance of objective feedback to accurate self-appraisal and use it effectively to make changes and build capacity. This Tier 2 group is designed for students who present with occupational challenges or positive screening difficulties related to: • Difficulty persisting in challenging tasks because they are striving for perfection • Being fearful of peer rejection or making mistakes at school • Viewing feedback as failure

	• Setting unrealistic goals
	• Acting confrontational or dismissively with others when constructive feedback provided
	• Becoming argumentative after making a mistake
	• Difficulty accepting personal responsibility
	• Inaccurately appraising one's abilities and competence in school activities
SESSION GOALS	1. Set up and complete several racetracks while blindfolded. 2. Discuss how feedback helped performance in this activity. 3. Consider how feedback from others may help with recent school performance issues. 4. Identify the process for forming new habits that help reframe points of feedbac objectively and minimize the impact of thinking traps on school performance.
OCCUPATION AS MEANS AND ENDS	Students participate in a leisure remote control car race to explore how feedback fr others can be helpful for improving personal causation and forming new habits to improve school performance.
DIRECTIONS	Students are given an opportunity to race remote control cars and learn the basic features of the car and remote. Once students are familiar with the tools, they select two racers who are blindfolded. The other students create an obstacle course. Grou members have to provide in-the-moment feedback to the racers so they can correc stay on track. The first racer to get to the finish line without going off track is the winner of that round. Repeat so each participant has several opportunities to race with their **eyes off the road**.
MATERIALS	• Two remote control race cars (batteries or chargers as required) • Two blindfolds or ways to occlude vision (turn around from the track) • Objects to create barriers or roadblocks and create the outline for the racetrack (tape, plastic cups, cones, foam pieces)
MESSY FACTOR	Medium
PINTEREST TERMS	Toy car racetrack, DIY kid racetrack, remote control car games
GRADE LEVEL	Middle and high schools

essing the Group: Tip Sheet

troduction and Warm-Up Ideas

scuss the differences between feedback and criticism

ve them look up and discuss the principles of carefrontation and review examples that distinguish *care-*
ntation from *con*frontation

ork through a feedback example to support problem setting (external to the person) and problem-solving
ategies that help to resolve the problem

ays to Grade or Modify the Activity

onsider if an audio or video recording replay may help students remember what was said and/or how racers
sponded to feedback

iminate the competition between two racers

ave racers turn around if they do not want to use a blindfold

sk the group to provide feedback to only one racer and not the other one to potentially reinforce the value
feedback more strongly

uestions You May Want to Ask

what instances and ways was feedback needed to race effectively? How might receiving feedback help
udents make changes that improve their performance on school tasks?

hat qualities of the feedback seemed most helpful to performing best? What made some aspects of feed-
ck less helpful?

hat tends to be the feedback you most frequently hear at school? How do you usually interpret that
edback?

ow do you normally process feedback on your performance at school? What changes, if any, can you make
process feedback in more helpful and healthy ways?

hat other things do you notice happen in your life when you respond negatively to feedback at school or
om people at school?

low skillful do you consider yourself to be at giving others feedback? What have been some challenges for
ou? What strategies could help you move away from confrontation and toward carefrontation with others?

hat change(s) do you see for yourself after participating in this activity?

acilitation Strategies

rovide examples of how feedback supported positive performance changes

rovide an example of working through feedback (e.g., picking out the parts that are objective, offer a helpful
trategy or solution)

iscuss different habits that may be useful for working through feedback

Facilitator's Notes

- Ways that feedback impacted volition (personal causation, self-efficacy, interests)

- Habits that reinforced negative outcomes and decreased performance

- Role of feedback for adaptation and improved participation at school

Group #26

Meghan Suman, OTD, OTR/L, BCP, SCSS

GROUP TITLE	Mixed Emotions
ACTIVITY	Game
PURPOSE	This group intervention focuses on emotional regulation and working through situations when one might feel a lot of different or **mixed emotions** at school. This group invites participants to play an emoji/emotion guessing game and to consider how different emotions impact behaviors and activity choices at school, especially some of those that have led to unfavorable consequences. The social nature of the group provides opportunities to naturally address self-awareness and social awareness in the context of real-life situations. Playing a social game also provides students with an opportunity to practice regulating emotions and following the rules, which can be highlighted when processing the group together.

This Tier 2 group may be helpful for students with occupational challenges and who have been identified by screening measures as struggling with:

- Being verbally aggressive or having confrontation with peers and teachers

- Facing peer rejection

- Having limited or no social participation

- Getting in trouble for acting out

- Following classroom and school rules

- Participating in school situations inappropriately and/or inconsistently because of being overwhelmed with negative or **mixed emotions** (guilt, shame, inadequacy, fear)

SESSION GOALS	1. Play the emoji game.
	2. Reinforce emotional literacy and encourage them to name emotions that were not in the game that can be tricky to understand and talk about.
	3. Highlight skills that reflect good use of self-regulation strategies while playing the game and processing the group.
	4. Consider the application of those skills to improve managing one's emotions at school.
OCCUPATION AS MEANS AND ENDS	This group uses a game activity to practice managing one's emotions while planning to make different activity and behavior choices at school when feeling **emotionally overwhelmed/mixed**.
DIRECTIONS	Each player selects a headband and adjusts it accordingly. **Mix up the emotions** by shuffling them on the table or floor face down. Players select one card (an emoji face), and without looking, clip it to their headband. The person with the birthday closest to Friendship Day (the first Sunday in August) tries to guess the emoji on the headband first. Each player has 1 minute to ask the group questions to which they are only able to provide facial expressions to indicate a **yes, maybe, no, or not sure** response. Questions will likely take the general form of "Is this a face I might make or an emotion I would feel if …" Players may not ask direct questions like, "What emoji is on my head?" or "Is the mouth turned up or down?" When a player is ready to guess the emoji on their headband, they will ask, "Am I [mimic the expression]?" (i.e., they will frown to suggest they have a frowning emoji). Each player who followed all the rules successfully that round will earn a chip. Players who did not follow the rules are encouraged to get a chip the next round. If all players earned a chip for that round, then the entire team gets a point. Individual prizes and team prizes are to be negotiated and determined by the group facilitator. Feel free to eliminate this aspect of the game if it does not fit therapeutically and just play for fun!
MATERIALS	• Headbands (an easy craft to make with paper and tape)
	• Paperclips to secure the emoji to the band
	• Emoji game tiles that can be made with open-source emojis (https://openmoji.org)
	• Possible prizes for winning player(s) or team(s)
MESSY FACTOR	Low
PINTEREST TERMS	Emoji games, headbands game DIY, DIY emoji activities
GRADE LEVEL	Elementary school

ole Emoji Cards

nages are taken from open-source platforms, but consider having participants draw their own!

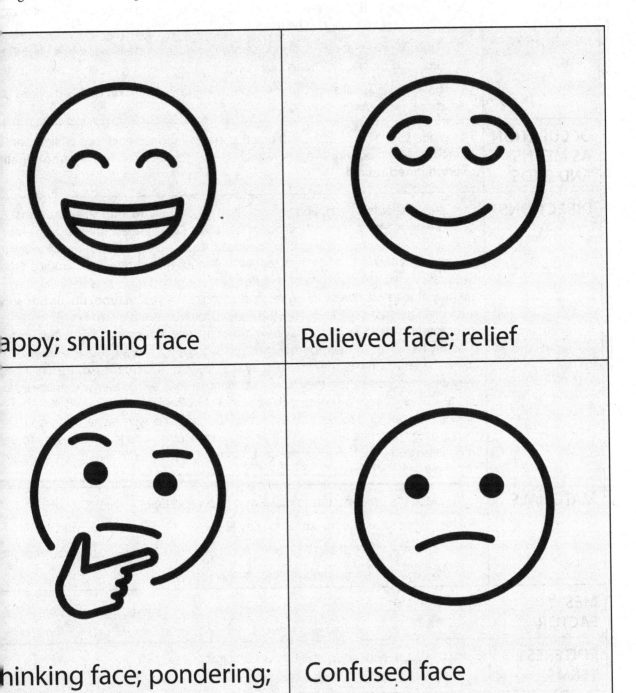

appy; smiling face

Relieved face; relief

hinking face; pondering;
uestioning

Confused face

Anxious face with sweat; worry

Angry face; mad

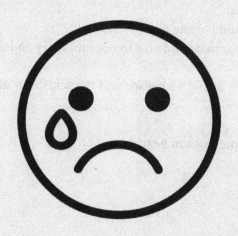

Sad face; crying; tears

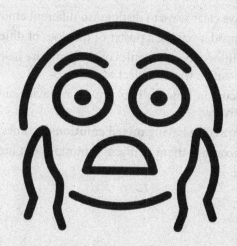

Scared; fear; fright

essing the Group: Tip Sheet

troduction and Warm-Up Ideas

·velop the group rules together since a major focus is on following rules and behavioral expectations

·eate a short story based on two or three emojis

This will help to ensure that they all understand and agree on the emotion

It might even be interesting to explore times when students share different emotions for the same emoji

·e how many different emotions the group can generate

·cognize a wide range of emotions is critical for emotional literacy

·ays to Grade or Modify the Activity

·ncourage students to draw or create their own emoji game pieces

·ld a role of referee to address any instances when rules are not followed or when there is a potential dispute

·out differences between similar but distinct emotions

·uestions You May Want to Ask

·hat kinds of things happen to you at school when your **emotions get mixed up** by life situations?

·hat activities can help you work through tough situations?

·hat activities could you do ahead of time to get yourself ready for challenging situations?

·ow can you make it a habit of checking in on yourself during the school day?

·ow do the classroom and school rules help us to figure out how to handle tough situations during the day?

·ow to manage your emotions during class activities?

·acilitation Strategies

·ave clear ways to distinguish different emotions for children

·onsider having a poster or handout of different emotions and healthy ways to respond

·einforce how the rules of the game are helping to know what to do and how to respond to try and develop

·positive way to reflect on rules

·ocus on how feelings impact behavior and our choices to or not to engage and participate in different

·ctivities

·ormalize having **mixed emotions** at times

·ncourage them to discuss emotions not included in the game that can be tricky

Facilitator's Notes

- How not being able to adapt emotionally limited meaningful participation and relationships

- Ways that occupations were discussed to build emotional strength

- Ways that occupations were discussed as a means to work through tough emotions

- Considerations for how to develop routines at school that might help them feel emotionally strong fo challenges that may arise

Group #27

Ashley Stoffel, OTD, OTR/L, FAOTA
and Lesly Wilson James, PhD, MPA, PMP, OTR/L, FAOTA

OUP TITLE	Brush It Off and Get It the Next Time
TIVITY	Cooking 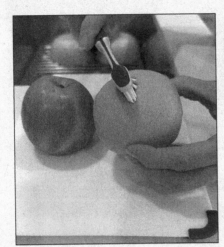 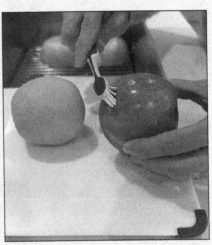
RPOSE	The purpose of this Tier 2 group is to support students in managing their emotions and expectations at school. The group encourages students to develop the habit of **brushing it off** after making mistakes and to explore how mistakes help us to learn and grow. During this group intervention, students use a soft toothbrush to literally **brush off** or clean fruit for a fruit salad. Facilitators intentionally draw students' attention to how their efforts of **brushing off** the fruit (and brushing it off again if it falls or rolls away) are positively supporting the collective goal of making a fruit salad. Students will be prompted to consider how **brushing off** frustration after making a mistake might help at school._x000D_
_x000D_
Occupationally well students are able to effectively adapt and adjust to changes at school. They persist in challenging tasks, learn from mistakes and feedback, and can revise their approaches so they can **get it the next time**._x000D_
_x000D_
This Tier 2 group may be most helpful to students who have positive screening results for the following occupational issues: • Worry about making mistakes • Avoid occupations that seem challenging at school • Judge their performance unrealistically • Experience shame and a sense of failure • Experience performance issues owing to a low sense of competence and limited expectations for school and academic success

	• Set goals and performance expectations too high • Difficulty coping to change(s) at school • Languish in self-criticism and perfectionism
SESSION GOALS	1. Clean fruit. 2. Make fruit salad. 3. Apply the **brush it off** metaphor to school situations.
OCCUPATION AS MEANS AND ENDS	This group uses a simple food preparatory/cooking task to encourage students to develop new habits around **brushing off** and learning from mistakes to perform better at school.
DIRECTIONS	The group members are presented with a simple recipe for a fruit kabob snack. Each member is handed a soft toothbrush to help them brush the dirt off the fruit before adding it to the bowl. Given the shape and size of the fruit (grapes, blueberries, strawberries), students are told that it is very likely some of the fruit will slip out of their hands and need to be brushed off. Each student is given a bowl of clean water to wash or brush the fruit off. When anyone drops a piece of fruit, the group says, **"It's okay. Just brush it off."** The group combines the clean fruit, serves it, and enjoys a healthy snack. The facilitator keeps a record of how often students **had to brush it** and reminds them that this strategy is supporting their efforts to make a fruit salad.
MATERIALS	• Soft toothbrushes (one for each group member) • Kid-safe skewers or thick straws • Small bowls (two for each group member) • Two bunches of grapes • One pint of blueberries • One pint of strawberries with stems removed • Paper towels or drying towels • Whipped topping or vanilla yogurt to dip fruit in (optional) • Clean water to wash fruit (Make sure to review any food allergies!)
MESSY FACTOR	Low to medium
PINTEREST TERMS	Kid-safe kabobs, fruit kabob recipes, fruit sparklers, homemade fruit and vegetable wash
GRADE LEVEL	Preschool and elementary schools

essing the Group: Tip Sheet

troduction and Warm-Up Ideas

are a social story about making mistakes and/or learning from mistakes
scuss how making healthy choices is good for our bodies and our minds (mental health)

ays to Grade or Modify the Activity

ve students serve each other
ry the recipe
corporate role play scenarios that might require **brushing off mistakes** at school

uestions You May Want to Ask

ow did having to start over or rewash a piece of fruit help you to make sure that everyone was eating clean uit? (Without fixing the mistake, we would be eating dirty fruit ... YUCK!)
hy was it easy to **brush it off** in this activity? What makes it hard to **brush it off** in other activities at school?
hat things did you do well in this activity? Why did it not matter that some fruit had to be rewashed?
ow safe did you feel in this activity to make a mistake without worrying about consequences? How safe do
u feel at school to make mistakes?
ow can doing the things we are good at help us get ourselves ready for doing things that are challenging and
ay require us to practice and try again?
ow does trying again and again lead to success?
hat do you think will help you use the **brush it off** strategy the next time you make a mistake at school?

acilitation Strategies

onsider participating in the activity yourself and highlight your own inevitable mistakes and the ease in
hich you **just brush it off**
einforce the benefits of learning from mistakes
ormalize that everyone makes mistakes and how they support learning and growth
rovide a lot of support/praise when they persist by brushing off the fruit again

Facilitator's Notes

- Factors that make students feel safe to make an error or mistake

- How activity encourages new habit formation

- School experiences that have been hard to **brush off** or **get it the next time**

- Self-imposed activity or occupation restrictions owing to perfectionism

- How metaphor applied to school

Group #28

Molly Bathje, PhD, MS, OTR/L

GROUP TITLE	Hidden Treasures
ACTIVITY	Treasure/scavenger hunt

PURPOSE	This group uses a **treasure** (scavenger) **hunt** activity to better understand how the physical and social environment of the school impacts the student in doing what they want and need to do. The group thinks about ways to make use of aspects of the environment (physical or social) that are supportive and problem solve around those that make things more challenging. As students work through and process the activity, they are expected to begin identifying how they might be able to use the **hidden treasures** at school to increase their overall satisfaction with going to school.

A positive school climate is linked to many factors that influence a student's mental health. Conversely, a negative school climate is often linked to factors like bullying and violence, which increases the risk of developing a mental illness and suicide. Occupationally successful students often describe their schools as safe and supportive places where they have been successful configuring and reconfiguring the spaces and relationships to develop themselves academically and to successfully meet student role expectations.

The group may be helpful for students who are languishing in an environment that may not support some of their respective occupational needs and who **do not**:

- Want to go to school
- Feel the school or classroom is safe
- Feel close to others or a sense of belonging at school
- Have opportunities to explore their personal interests at school
- Have a sense of being able to control outcomes or events at school
- Have routine social interactions that are positive and supportive
- Have coping strategies to leverage the school environment
- Fully participate in school activities and student role
- Take advantage of social opportunities at school

SESSION GOALS	1. Complete the treasure hunt. 2. Reinforce the possibility for the small group experiences to provide supportive social interactions. 3. Consider different coping strategies that might make the student perceive the school environment more positively. 4. Consider environmental modifications that might make the student perceive the school environment more positively.
OCCUPATION AS MEANS AND ENDS	This group uses a treasure hunt activity to consider ways to change the student–school environment fit to improve participation.
DIRECTIONS	The facilitator prints off a treasure map for each participant. The students review each question on the map and begin to generate ideas about how to answer the question. The facilitator asks students to share some of the places they have identified and makes a list of the places students identified. The group then visits each of the spaces on the list generated by the group, along with additional spaces identified by the facilitator. As the group moves together throughout the school, students consider if each of the spaces visited fits on their treasure map and record their answers on the map. After walking the school grounds for 30 minutes (time could vary greatly), the facilitator can lead group processing by having each student share their unique map and discuss why they chose the spaces they did. The group can also process how many clues they did not answer and what was difficult about finding an answer for those clues, how many students answered clues similarly, and what aspects of the person–environment fit may be lacking for each student in the group. All the clues had the "student" in common. The big question of the group is: **How could it be possible that finding the hidden treasures at school could help discover some of the hidden treasures within themselves?**

	Example spaces include:
	- Homeroom
	- Library
	- Art room
	- Music room
	- Gymnasium
	- Lunch room
	- Nurse's office
	- Principal's office
	- School social worker/counselor's office
	- Occupational therapy/speech-language pathology/physical therapy space
	- Bathroom
	- Stairwells
	- Lockers
	- Playground
	- Parking lot
	- Exterior spaces with trees, shrubs, or flowers
	- Art displays
ATERIALS	- Treasure map with person–environment clues or questions
	- Pencils
	- Art materials (if you decorate the treasure maps)
ESSY CTOR	Low
NTEREST RMS	Treasure hunt clue cards for kids, treasure map template, treasure map coloring page, easy DIY pirate patch for kids, classroom treasure chest ideas
RADE VEL	Elementary school

Treasures (at School) Map

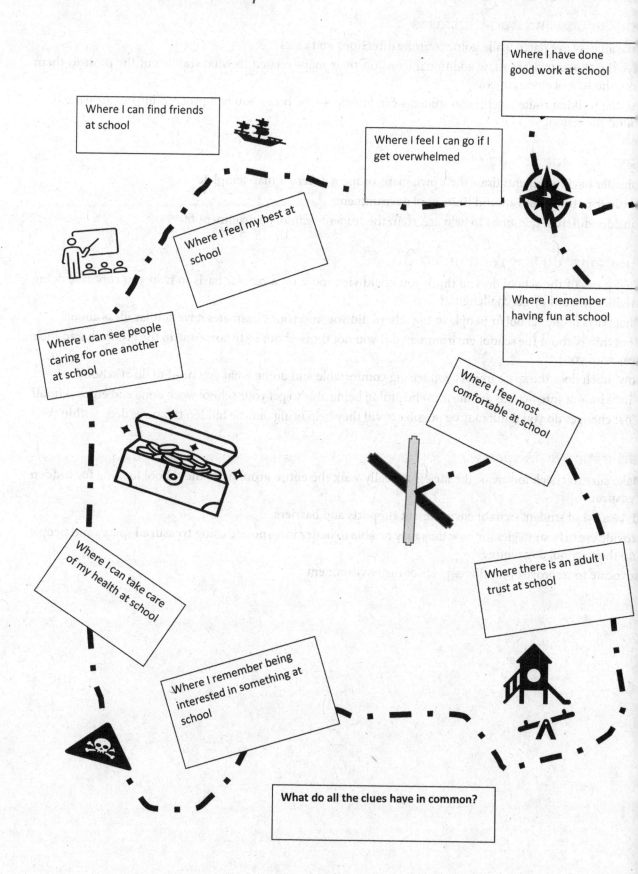

Where I can find friends at school

Where I have done good work at school

Where I feel I can go if I get overwhelmed

Where I feel my best at school

Where I remember having fun at school

Where I can see people caring for one another at school

Where I feel most comfortable at school

Where I can take care of my health at school

Where there is an adult I trust at school

Where I remember being interested in something at school

What do all the clues have in common?

essing the Group: Tip Sheet

troduction and Warm-Up Ideas

ake an easy eye patch while going over the directions and clues

ive the students draw a few additional icons on their maps related to what stands out the most to them out the school environment

an the walking route together so students can anticipate the order you will proceed in your treasure hunt und the school

ays to Grade or Modify the Activity

onsider having students draw their own maps or use a different map template

onsider putting clues around the school environment

onsider different questions to help ascertain the student–school environment fit

uestions You May Want to Ask

hat parts of the school do you think you could visit more on a regular basis to help you continue doing tivities when they get challenging?

hat parts of the school or people in the school did you and your classmates have similar ideas about?

hat things about the school environment did you not think about until someone in the group shared their eas with you?

ow much does the space impact you feeling comfortable and doing what you need to do at school?

hat kinds of interactions are the most helpful in being able to get your school work done and enjoy school?

hat changes do you think may be possible? Will they help bring out the hidden treasures deep within you?

acilitation Strategies

ake sure to check footwear; the idea is to really walk the entire grounds of the school looking for **hidden easures**

ake a list of student–school environment supports and barriers

rovide creative strategies for how they may be able to better incorporate using **treasured** spaces and people to their school day routine

dvocate to improve or modify aspects of the environment

Facilitator's Notes

- Spaces that seem to support school participation

- Recurring misfits between student–school environment

- Adaptations or modifications to make environment more safe or positive

Group #29

*Karen Stornello, OTD, OTR/L
and Renee Harris, COTA/L*

OUP TITLE	Wii Means **WE**
TIVITY	Setting up a gaming system and playing video games

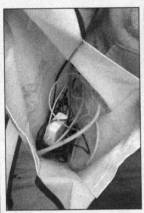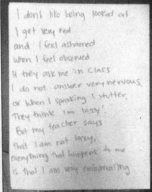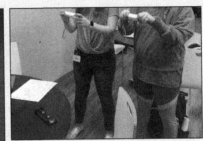

RPOSE

This small group intervention requires students to figure out how to connect different parts of a game console to the television so they can play video games. This therapeutic group requires students to literally determine what pieces, parts, and steps are needed to connect the game console and television together. Students are prompted to consider the process metaphorically and determine what pieces, parts, and steps may be useful in changing habits of doing things in a solitary manner to new habits of doing with others and intentionally trying to build social connections at school. The group then examines how adding more **"we"** experiences into one's routine may support increased pride, connection, and opportunities to get out of the cycle of shame.

The group may be helpful for students who are languishing socially and may tend to:

- Experience negative emotions (e.g., worry, dread, incompetence) when interacting with peers
- Not feel confident or worthy of attention or support from others
- Use self-deprecating statements to encourage disconnection from others so activities can be done in isolation
- Feel shame and possibly shame others to feel better in occupations involving social interactions
- Not expect to do things well so they do not try new things or push self to engage in things that will build skill

SESSION GOALS	1. Connect the gaming system to the television or monitor.
	2. Discuss opportunities to build stronger social connections at school using occupations and personal interests.
	3. Play video games together.
OCCUPATION AS MEANS AND ENDS	Using a gamified leisure challenge to connect a Wii (Nintendo) gaming console syst to a television and the internet to help students develop a plan for participating in more social activities and building stronger social connections at school.
DIRECTIONS	In this group activity, students literally have to explore the steps and the equipmen needed to set up a Wii gaming device and control a television or monitor. This task is done using a gamified approach, because the group will have to answer question (shame quiz questions included) about how shame shows up in our everyday lives order to select a box. Each box contains cords and adaptors or information that will either be helpful or of no value to connecting the Wii system. Players will likely beg to recognize that certain pieces help with connection whereas other pieces do not. This figurative point is discussed later when processing the activity and how it appli to moving beyond shame. Eventually, the group obtains all the required instruction: and cords they need to successfully get the Wii up and running so they can actually play a few rounds of games.
MATERIALS	• Wii gaming system and controllers
	• Television
	• Wii games
	• Instructions to connect the console to the television and the internet (maybe ha pictures or visual aids)
	• Distractor or unnecessary cords, adaptors, directions, and tools
MESSY FACTOR	Low
PINTEREST TERMS	Toxic shame, empathy, empathy word cloud, shame vs. guilt, daring classrooms
GRADE LEVEL	Middle and high schools

ne *Quiz Questions*

h of the questions, ask the group members to consider whether they agree, disagree, or are not sure. You
vant to give each member a card with each option written on it and they can hold up their responses. These
some **suggested questions** that explore the occupational impact of shame.

ry to avoid activities that will cause me to have to talk about my feelings.

vill make jokes about myself to cover up my mistakes when I am not doing something well.

hen I do not perform well, I get angry with myself or with other people.

is easier to criticize my performance than it is to recognize my strengths and skills.

end to be so serious that other people do not enjoy my company.

vould rather do things by myself than risk being humiliated by other people.

is easier to engage superficially with other people than to risk being vulnerable.

lo not really have any relaxing activities in my routine because I do not want to disappoint others or appear
zy.

want to do things my way, which usually limits how often I have to work with others.

do things that are not always healthy when I am angry or feeling shame.

know how to remove shame from my self-talk or feedback to others.

know activities that allow me or would help me practice self-compassion.

try really hard to do things perfectly.

Agree

Disagree

Not Sure

Let's talk some more

essing the Group: Tip Sheet

troduction and Warm-Up Ideas

are examples of things in everyday life we must connect to (Wi-Fi, power, one end to another, router, Zoom eeting)

view different quotes about shame and discuss what seems to resonate most

are a short poem about shame and have a quick discussion

actice removing shame from statements (e.g., "I'm a loser" vs. "I lost the game")

ays to Grade or Modify the Activity

onsider answering the shame quiz questions anonymously to make students feel less vulnerable

t the students use resources and technology to find a video on how to set up the gaming system and sup- rting connection cords

uestions You May Want to Ask

atures of the cord and the console had to fit to establish a connection. What kinds of things must fit to nnect with others?

hen the items were disconnected, they have very little use to anyone. How does being disconnected at times terfere with being able to meet expectations positively?

hat activities might offer you a way to feel more connected at school?

hat do you feel you need to change your habits that disconnect you to ones that connect you with others?

hat kinds of activities can you put into your routine to feel more pride and less shame?

his group turned an activity that is usually done alone into a **we** activity. What activities do you normally do one that could be enriched by doing it with other people? What opportunities do you see for making social nnections stronger by just using your personal interests?

ow might you be able to use feedback from others whom you trust to help you anticipate successful utcomes?

hat situations might get better for you at school if you do activities that help you work through shame?

hat things does shame keep you from doing?

acilitation Strategies

e explicit about the group being a safe space and expectations of confidentiality

einforce regularly that it took "we" to get the Wii up and running

e mindful of how students respond to the quiz questions so you can return to it

emind them of cords and contents that were useless to connecting the Wii as a way to consider habits and ays of doing that might be fostering disconnection rather than connection

Facilitator's Notes

- Group behaviors that supported inclusion and connection

- How occupation encouraged participation and supported self-efficacy

- Ways you used yourself therapeutically to foster connection

- How group cohesion advanced during the activity

- How you processed what was happening in the actual group with what you suspect may happen at times or in other contexts during the school day

Group #30

Erin Schwier, EdD, OTD, OTR/L

GROUP TITLE	Rough Seas: Riding the Waves or Going Overboard
ACTIVITY	Craft

PURPOSE	This therapeutic group invites students to complete a craft activity and identify thinking traps that may be increasing their anxiety or feelings of dread and worry a[t] school. Specifically, the group explores how students may have habits associated w[ith] catastrophizing situations and not expecting successful outcomes. The goal is to he[lp] them look at thinking traps, practice more accurately appraising the size of problem[s] and improve their volition so they are more willing to engage in new tasks more confidently at school. The group may be helpful for students who are languishing emotionally and may tend to: • Be highly self-critical and have an inaccurate sense of abilities • Have performance struggles owing to excessive worrying and feeling ineffectiv[e] • Feel a heightened sense of dread in otherwise ordinary situations • Expect negative outcomes • Make activity choices based on a strong fear of failure • Consider all change to be bad and attempt to avoid it • Give up easily when faced with a challenge they quickly label as impossible
SESSION GOALS	1. Make a craft. 2. Apply a new cognitive strategy to minimize tendency to catastrophize. 3. Identify ways to develop new habits.
OCCUPATION AS MEANS AND ENDS	Using a craft activity to encourage students to consider new habits and performanc[e] patterns that could help them persist confidently in school tasks/situations that are challenging.
DIRECTIONS	**Phase 1:** Students are asked to build a craft stick raft using the available supplies provided. The facilitator encourages the participants to brainstorm some designs initially. After a few minutes, the group is provided with instructions for different raft patterns to review. Not providing explicit patterns encourages brainstorming and problem solving. It also allows the facilitator to observe if anyone sees not having a template as a "big," frustrating problem. If so, this can be processed later in the discussion. It is recommended that 15 minutes be provided to brainstorm and construct the raft. This increases the likelihood that the glue can dry. **Phase 2:** Students sail their rafts. Each student places their boat in the water bath and gives it a nudge. Once the boat is in the water, they are instructed not to pull it out. However, they are encouraged to try and save their boat from sinking, if possible[.] The goal is to have their boat sail to the finish line without falling apart or sinking. It i[s] recommended to consider 10 minutes for this phase of the activity.

TERIALS	• Several craft sticks • White school glue (water soluble, such as Elmer's [Newell Rubbermaid]) • Tape • Paper • Embellishments (stickers, glitter, sequins) • Scissors • Markers • Paper (for sails) • Styrofoam pieces (optional) • Clear plastic tote, basin, or cooler to fill with water to sail rafts on • Towels to wipe up any spills
SSY CTOR	Low to medium
NTEREST RMS	Popsicle boat, stick raft, popsicle stick boat craft, floating craft for kids, easy pouring station, DIY water table
ADE VEL	Middle school

Sample Instructions for Basic Popsicle Raft

There are several online you may want to print out for review. Encourage creativity and varied designs.

1. Line up three or four popsicle sticks horizontally with a little gap between each stick

2. Squeeze a line of glue along each stick and then place vertical sticks to create the base of the raft.

3. Near the middle of the raft, leave a small space between two vertical sticks so you can place the sail between the raft boards.

4. Make the sail by using a single stick and attaching a paper triangle. Consider decorating the sail with something that represents one of your strengths or something you value.

5. Decorate and embellish your raft. Have fun!

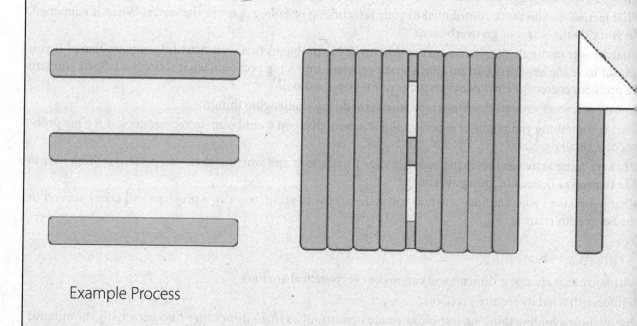

Example Process

essing the Group: Tip Sheet

troduction and Warm-Up Ideas

are examples of small, medium, and big problems at school or in everyday life

ow students pictures of common items that have been magnified out of proportion and see if they can ess what they are; keep a record of how many guesses it takes

are an example of when someone (maybe yourself) thought something was a big problem when it was tually only a small problem

ays to Grade or Modify the Activity

not provide any instructions for how to construct the raft

ve less time for construction so the glue is less dry

ave small, medium, big, and jumbo craft sticks available in different quantities

ve students a second chance to fix their rafts and have a successful second sail

ave students swap rafts halfway through the activity

ovide students with a set of materials and instruct them to use all the pieces

uestions You May Want to Ask

hat was challenging about completing this activity for you?

hat factors do you think contributed to your raft sinking or falling apart in the water? When it happened, d you ride the waves or **go overboard**?

hat aspects of the challenge did you consider to be big problems that were actually small problems? If you d not have the experience of turning a small problem into a big problem, what strategies helped you size e problem correctly? How does this play out for you at school?

ow do you work around thinking traps when you do try challenging things?

hat is something you might be experiencing at school that you would want to reconsider if it is a big probm or a small problem?

hat are some activities that help you settle your frustrations and worries when you need to rethink how to de the waves instead of going overboard?

hat happens to your confidence when you rethink how to accurately size a problem and take a second or ird or fourth chance?

acilitation Strategies

ormalize that change is difficult and can make everyone feel anxious

einforce that habits require practice

iscuss how avoiding thinking traps may create opportunities to do things they find personally meaningful

einforce the role of making mistakes with learning new things

e intentional about having group members support one another

Facilitator's Notes

- Student behaviors that suggested frustration/catastrophizing

- How occupation encouraged participation and supported self-efficacy

- Ways you used yourself therapeutically to encourage coping with changing circumstances

- How group members supported each other during the activity and discussion

- How you processed what was happening in the actual group with what you suspect may happen at times or in other contexts during the school day

Group #31

*Sarah Nielsen, PhD, OTR/L, FAOTA; Bobbi Carrlson, PhD, OTR/L;
and Janet S. Jedlicka, PhD, OTR/L, FAOTA*

OUP TITLE	Partying While Party Planning
TIVITY	Game and party planning
RPOSE	The purpose of this group is to support students who do not have a strong sense of belonging at school to participate in socially meaningful activities. The group is designed so that participants complete a **party planning** project as they **party while they party plan**. The game also challenges students who do not feel like they fit in to play around with making ideas fit in with a theme provided on a game card. The idea of a party was chosen because they are occupations in which bonding and connecting can occur naturally. The **party planning game** presents scenarios and challenges that require teamwork, interest exploration, and help to brainstorm ideas for the party they are eventually responsible for hosting. As such, the group challenge provides them with an opportunity to become a **party planning committee**. Secondarily, the group gives students the opportunity to reimagine their school as a space where meaningful relationships can be built through doing activities together. Consider this small group intervention when the problem-solving team has student concerns about the following occupational issues at school: • Avoiding social interactions with others during school activities owing to low self-confidence • Lacking a sense of belonging to a peer group • Lacking self-esteem • Not being sure how to fit in with a group • Having difficulty connecting with others at school • Restricting oneself to activity choices that are mostly solitary in nature • Feeling anxious or increased worry when having to interact with peers for school tasks (e.g., group projects, finding people to each lunch with, building friendships)

SESSION GOALS	1. Students play a game about **party planning**.
	2. Students are assigned the role of being a member of a **party planning committee**.
	3. Students use the ideas generated in the game to host a future party at school.
OCCUPATION AS MEANS AND ENDS	Using a game about party planning to build meaningful social interactions and explore fitting in while also assigning the role of **party planning committee** member to encourage them to actually plan and host a party.
DIRECTIONS	Students will play a team-based game designed to practice **party planning** tasks while fostering interaction and a sense of connection and fitting in. Gameplay occurs in three rounds. Round 1 starts after a player flips over a party theme card from the stack. Each team gets 5 minutes to plan a snack that is associated with the theme. Each team presents their idea to the group, and then the group votes on the best snack idea based on how well it fits in with the theme and how simple, inexpensive, nutritious, and easy it is to make at school. For round 2, each team gets 5 minutes to brainstorm a fun party activity related to the theme. Each team votes on the best activity idea based on goodness of fit with the theme and how well it matches collective interests and seems fun. Round 3 involves the teams in planning a party favor based on the theme and voting on the best one based on fit with theme, cost, and simplicity. Each winning idea earns the team a point. The team with the greatest number of points gets to pick the theme for a class party. All group members then organize and host the party in a few weeks. Essentially, they leverage these connections to become a **party planning committee**.
	Each round focuses on how well the idea fits in with the theme to provide space for you to discuss the occupational struggles associated with fitting in at school. Because the game is designed to help players connect and develop camaraderie, we encourage you to keep playing until you begin to see signs of connection and a team spirit emerging.
	(There are so many occupations you can incorporate into group activities as the group gets ready to throw and host the party!)
MATERIALS	· A stack of party theme cards
	· Student handout or checklist on being part of a team (optional)
	· Writing surface for keeping score and collecting ideas
	· Instrument for keeping time (e.g., stopwatch, phone, timer, hourglass)
MESSY FACTOR	Low
PINTEREST TERMS	Teamwork infographic, classroom party, party theme, cheap party favors, teambuilding, inclusion
GRADE LEVEL	Elementary and middle schools

Theme Card Examples

pular movies	Holidays	Music	Big surprises
World events	Popular memes	Acts of kindness	Sports
Books	Camping	Comic books	TV shows
mous women	Careers	Trains, planes, and autos	Wild card

ke the mood fun and partylike. There are no correct or incorrect answers. Encourage creativity! They will
e learning about each other through playing the game. Remember, the focus should be on bonding and
ting and fitting in with one another.

ow is a possible example to help jumpstart the game or to help illustrate the rules:
e theme card "Books" is chosen. One team gets excited by *How to Eat Fried Worms*.
und 1: They offer the idea of a gummy worm snack served in a French fry container
und 2: They think it would be fun to do the worm dance (breakdancing)
und 3: They suggest making bookworm bookmarks for everyone

essing the Group: Tip Sheet

troduction and Warm-Up Ideas

nare past experiences of party activities that seemed to get everyone involved
nare a quote about inclusion or belonging and have them reflect
xplore what fitting in and connecting with others looks like at school

Vays to Grade or Modify the Activity

ave the students generate the party theme cards
et the students use resources and technology to help them come up with ideas
lay as one team and just vote the best or most creative ideas each round

Questions You May Want to Ask

What were some of the strategies that either you or a group member used to offer a sense of belonging?
How did having a shared activity help you feel connected to each other?
What might change for you if you begin to feel more connected at school?
What changes can be made to make the school environment more inclusive and help everyone fit in better?
How might strategies experienced today be useful in other ways at school?
What school situations might get better for you at school if it becomes easier to feel like you fit in?
What supports might you need to do the tasks associated with being a member of the **party planning
ommittee**?
How might doing this role well give you an opportunity to make an impact on your school socially? What
ind of meaning do you imagine that might have for you?

Facilitation Strategies

Keep track of winning ideas each round and reflect back how all the students contributed to overall party ideas
Ask students to brainstorm how to make the atmosphere more partylike (e.g., put on some music, get
comfortable)
Ask about behaviors they saw in themselves and you that supported a sense of inclusion and belonging

Facilitator's Notes

- Observe and document children's capacity for cooperation and creativity

- Consider therapeutic use of self-strategies that foster children solving conflict

- Observe how the self-efficacy of each child grew during the experience

Group #32

Cindy Sears, OTD, MA, OTR/L, BCP

GROUP TITLE	Feeling the Heat and Keeping Your Cool
ACTIVITY	Cooking
PURPOSE	The primary purpose of this cooking activity is to explore the extent to which students perceive their school environment challenges their ability to **stay cool** when stressful situations occur or when things **heat up at school**. In particular, the group members are encouraged to examine the ways in which the consequences of **not keeping their cool** has had on their ability to fully participate at school and get satisfaction from going to school. The cooking group literally examines how foods and ingredients respond to heat in ways that benefit the recipe and metaphorically encourage each student to commit to behaving more adaptively (i.e., **keeping their cool**) when they **feel the heat from school**. Group members also consider possible modifications to the environment that could strengthen their commitment to change and expectation for successful outcomes.
	Occupationally well students use the classroom and school rules, as well as social expectations, to make activity and behavioral choices that comply with guidelines. They demonstrate effective self-regulation and have habits that support them in being able to think before they act. They are also able to effectively incorporate strategies into their school routine that help them **stay cool** when school situations **amp up the heat**.

	The group may be helpful for students who are languishing emotionally and experience the following occupational concerns owing to externalizing and internalizing behaviors: • Exhibit emotional outbursts in class that cause disruptions to self and other learners • Have difficulty standing up for themselves in challenging situations • Feel overwhelmed by school tasks • Feel a large amount of stress and anxiety at school • Break school and classroom rules • Have difficulty coping/adapting to changes at school
SESSION GOALS	1. Make a lunch together requiring a heat source. 2. Evaluate how different ingredients changed favorably in the presence of a heat source. 3. Identify situations and times during the school day when the **heat is up** and commit to new ways of responding favorably to the **heat**.
OCCUPATION AS MEANS AND ENDS	Using a cooking activity to build skills and habits around self-regulation and encourage activity choices that better meet the expectations of the environment and student role.
DIRECTIONS	This activity provides students with an opportunity to make a lunch together. The menu for this small group intervention is pasta and garlic toast, and the three ingredients serve as the metaphor for group processing: pasta, salt, and bread. Each of these ingredients responds differently to the heat in a somewhat opposite manner: the pasta goes from hard to soft, the bread goes from soft to hard, and the salt goes from visible to invisible. These changes metaphorically invite students to consider how it might be beneficial for them to behave in ways or participate in activities that support going from **feeling heated to keeping their cool**. The activity also highlights the benefits of the heat source to the individual ingredients (i.e., the spaghetti is not edible without the hot water) and encourages the students metaphorically explore if some of the **heat** they feel at school helps them realize the purpose more fully.

TERIALS	• Kettle or hot plate • Toaster • Large pot with lid • Knife and utensils • Plates • Colander • Pasta • Pasta sauce and topping • Water • Bread • Butter or spread • Salt • Garlic seasoning (Be mindful of any dietary restrictions and modify the recipe accordingly.)
ESSY CTOR	High
NTEREST RMS	Cooking experiments, legit meals in the microwave, toaster garlic bread, microwave spaghetti, toaster oven meals
RADE VEL	Middle and high schools

THE PARABLE OF THE CARROT, THE EGG, AND THE COFFEE BEAN AT SCHOOL

A teacher was discussing adversity with her students. The students shared stories of life being challenging and difficult. To encourage more thinking, the teacher filled three small bowls with water. the first bowl, she placed some fresh baby carrots. In the second bowl, she placed an egg. In the third bowl, she added a few coffee beans. After putting them in the microwave on high for 4 minutes, the teacher took them out and let them cool for a few minutes.

The teacher asked the students, "Tell me, class, what do you see?"

One student replied, "There are carrots, an egg, and coffee."

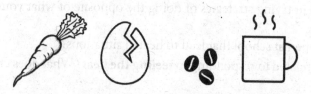

The teacher then had the students pass the cooled bowls around and feel the carrots, break one of the eggs, and smell the coffee. A few students noted the carrots had turned soft. Other students observed that the eggs had hardened and it helped to peel the shells. Another student replied that the coffee smelled good and asked the teacher, "What do these foods have to do with adversity?"

The teacher explained that each of the foods had faced the same adversity: being placed in boiling hot water. Each also reacted differently. The teacher explained that the carrots went from hard strong, and tough to becoming soft and mushy. The egg, which was originally very fragile with a very thin skin, became hardened after being in the hot water. Lastly, the coffee beans were a bit unique Rather than changing themselves, the coffee beans changed the water once it came to a boil.

The teacher asked the students, "Which are you?" She reiterated by asking, "When adversity come knocking on your door, are you a carrot, an egg, or a coffee bean?"

Adapted for the school setting. Original author unknown.

essing the Group: Tip Sheet

troduction and Warm-Up Ideas

ve students review the carrot, the egg, and the coffee bean story (provided)

ite the students to consider situations when opposite action strategies can help (doing the opposite of at you think your emotions are telling you to do)

view some opposite action skills associated with dialectical behavior therapy

ays to Grade or Modify the Activity

ter the recipe in ways to make it easier or fit with supplies on hand

e the microwave as the primary heat source

cus on how one food or ingredient may respond to heat (e.g., popcorn)

uestions You May Want to Ask

hen have challenges with **keeping your cool** impacted school outcomes?

hat strengths and talents get overlooked when you are viewed as someone who cannot keep their cool?

ow might those strengths and talents support you in making different behavior choices at school?

hat benefits do you see in trying strategies of doing the opposite of what your emotions are telling you to ?

hat kinds of things happen at school that lead to heated situations?

hat habits do you have related to responding to **feeling the heat**? What does changing your habits look like r you?

hat activities have you noticed help you **keep your cool**?

what ways did the metaphors in this group apply to your situation at school? In what ways did they not ply?

fter this activity, what change can you commit to making at school? How will you measure success? What pports or resources do you need to make that change stick?

acilitation Strategies

ormalize that people respond to **heat** differently—just like the different ingredients

how how students' values and consequences are not aligned

einforce how the skills in perspective-taking during the group can be used to make different behavior hoices in the future

Facilitator's Notes

- The different perspectives that were taken and shared

- How consequences compromised participation in meaningful activities

- Ways in which the metaphor resonated with their school experiences

- Changes they hope to make and expected impact on occupational performance

Group #33

*Brad E. Egan, OTD, PhD, CADC, OTR/L
and Susan Cahill, PhD, OTR/L, FAOTA*

GROUP TITLE	Holding It All Together: Experimenting With Icing
ACTIVITY	Cooking/graham cracker candy houses

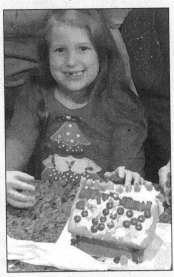 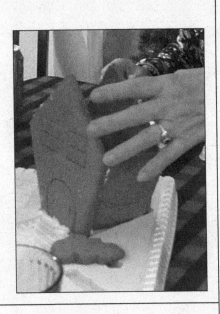

PURPOSE	The primary purpose of this creative cooking activity is to create an opportunity for students to identify a new "recipe" of behaviors and thoughts that could help them with **holding it all together** at school. The group invites participants to develop an icing recipe that serves as the glue for a graham cracker house. Group members have to evaluate how well the icing is **holding it all together** and modify the recipe accordingly.

The primary purpose of this creative cooking activity is to create an opportunity for students to identify a new "recipe" of behaviors and thoughts that could help them with **holding it all together** at school. The group invites participants to develop an icing recipe that serves as the glue for a graham cracker house. Group members have to evaluate how well the icing is **holding it all together** and modify the recipe accordingly.

Developing self-monitoring and self-management skills is important for staying motivated at school, managing impulses, complying with behavioral classroom expectations, and pursuing long-term educational goals. Students in this Tier 2 group discuss the successes and challenges associated with creating new habits that help with managing all the stressors, expectations, changes, and pressures that sometimes make it difficult to **hold it all together** at school.

The group may be helpful for students who are languishing personally and may tend to:

- Have difficulty self-regulating throughout the school day
- Have challenges following classroom and school rules
- Lack strategies for changing their behaviors or thoughts to meet academic goals
- Demonstrate limited success in organizing their environment to reduce stress
- Experience meltdowns or regular feelings of being overwhelmed
- Have difficulty or have stopped participating in personally meaningful school activities and relationships

SESSION GOALS	1. Create an icing recipe using the materials provided. 2. Use the icing to build a graham cracker house and evaluate how effectively it **holds it all together**. 3. Modify the recipe so the graham cracker house **holds together**. 4. Discuss how personal behaviors and thoughts (just like the icing recipe) can be modified at school to help with **holding it all together**. 5. Have participants share with each other what habits have helped them to mon and modify their behaviors and in what areas they still experience challenges.
OCCUPATION AS MEANS AND ENDS	This group uses the occupation of cooking, specifically creating a royal icing, to mal a graham cracker house and explore self-regulation strategies at school. As an ends students identify ways their approach to modifying their icing recipes may also hel them to develop habits that make it easier to **hold it all together** at school.
DIRECTIONS	Students individually use the provided ingredients and a process of trial and error to create a royal icing strong enough to hold a graham cracker house together. Students are given a blank recipe card and asked to write down modifications as the go along. The facilitator may provide hints along the way and/or encourage them to share different recipe ideas with one another. They are encouraged to decorate their individual houses and share the strategies that were most helpful in **holding it all together**. Lastly, the group discusses how developing new strategies and habits might help them to **hold it all together** better at school and support them in meeting their long-term academic goals.
MATERIALS	• A few bags of confectioners' or powdered sugar • Milk • Vanilla extract • Maple or corn syrup • Variety of hard candies • Sandwich or icing bags • Toothpicks • A few boxes of graham crackers • Plates and trays • Spatulas • Spoons
MESSY FACTOR	High
PINTEREST TERMS	Super sticky glue icing, simple gingerbread houses, holiday cuteness icing recipes, royal icing recipe
GRADE LEVEL	Middle school

essing the Group: Tip Sheet

troduction and Warm-Up Ideas

ve students select different decorations for their graham cracker candy house
scuss previous experiences with trial-and-error approaches and how they strategized

ays to Grade or Modify the Activity

ovide a recipe card with the ingredients but not the measurements
ake stable houses ahead of time and only have them try to secure candy and decorations
ve them brainstorm the recipe as a group

uestions You May Want to Ask

hat strategies did you come up with that helped you the most?
hat did you notice that helped you determine if your icing was strong enough to **hold it all together** or
t?
 what ways do you take notice of yourself during the school day to see if you are **holding it all together**
ell or not?
 what ways did sharing thoughts with other group members impact your recipe? Did it help? Do you think
at you discovered the right measurements faster because of their tips?
ow might sharing thoughts with others be a strategy for **holding it all together** at school better?
re there times when or places where it seems easy to **hold it all together**? If so, describe them.
re there times when or places where it seems difficult or messy to **hold it all together**? If so, describe them.
ow does this activity apply to some of the challenges you experience at school?
hat habits from this activity do you think could be used to help **hold it all together** better? How can you
se them during the school day?

acilitation Strategies

ormalize that it might take many attempts to develop a recipe strong enough to **hold it all together**
upport self-efficacy by allowing them to problem solve solutions that they feel may work for them
ake notice of the strategies and habits that are working well and intentionally share and reflect on those
hen processing the group
ncourage persistence by providing hints and support as needed

Facilitator's Notes

- Habits that were helpful to the project

- Qualities of spaces that seem to help with self-regulation

- School challenges that were discussed and described

- Strategies needed to keep participants engaged and persisting in the activity when it became difficult or they experienced setbacks (e.g., house feel apart, decorations fell off, it became too messy)

Section 4

Data Collection Tools

Egan, B. E., Sears, C., & Keener, A. (Eds.). *Occupational Therapy Groups for A*
Mental Health Challenges in School-Aged Populations: A Tier 2 Resource (pp. 2

   Data collection tools may also be used as screening tools for identifying students who would benef
mental health supports, as well as serving as pre- and post-data measurements to monitor student progre
time (Figures 4-1 through 4-7). These measures can be completed by the occupational therapist, school
istrators, guidance counselors, teachers, and even the student themselves when appropriate. The data co
tools are evidence-based ability maps derived from a Rasch analysis of standardized measures. These abilit
can be used to determine personalized student goals. They are ordered on the basis of difficulty, with the
item on the bottom and the hardest at the top.

Behavior Compliance
Data Tracking Form

Student Name:_____ School:_____ Date:_____ Skills Score %:_____

Instructions: The student receives a score of 1 for every expected behavior demonstrated. The score is determined as a percentage of behaviors demonstrated divided by behaviors expected. Item #1 is the easiest cooperative behavior to demonstrate and item #10 is the hardest cooperative behavior to demonstrate.

☐ 10. Raises hand to ask a question

☐ 9. Follows time limits set by adult

☐ 8. Cleans up at appropriate time

☐ 7. Observes rules regarding movement in hallways

☐ 6. Observes rules regarding bathroom use

☐ 5. Shows care in use and handling others' property

☐ 4. Stops when asked to do so

☐ 3. Observes class and school rules

☐ 2. Cooperates with requests

☐ 1. Proceeds as directed when told to begin

Figure 4-1. Behavior Compliance Data Tracking Form. (Adapted from Hwang, J. L., & Davies, P. L. [2009]. Rasch analysis of the School Function Assessment provides additional evidence for the internal validity of the activity performance scales. *American Journal of Occupational Therapy, 63*[3], 369-373, https://doi.org/10.5014/ajot.63.3.369)

CONFLICT RESOLUTION SKILLS DATA TRACKING FORM

Student Name:_____ School:_____

Date:_____ Skills Score %:_____

Instructions: The student receives a score of 1 for every skill demonstrated. The score is determined as a percentage of skills demonstrated divided by skills expected. Item #1 is the easiest skill to demonstrate and item #5 is the hardest skill to demonstrate.

☐ 5. Resolves ordinary conflict without requesting teacher assistance

☐ 4. Handles frustration when experiencing difficulties at school

☐ 3. Uses words rather than physical action to respond when angry

☐ 2. Maintains control of self in large groups

☐ 1. Accepts unexpected changes in routine

Figure 4-2. Conflict Resolution Skills Data Tracking Form. (Adapted from Hwang, J. L., & Davies, P. L. [2009]. Rasch analysis of the School Function Assessment provides additional evidence for the internal validity of the activity performance scales. *American Journal of Occupational Therapy, 63*[3], 369-373. https://doi.org/10.5014/ajot.63.3.369)

GROUP BEHAVIORS DATA TRACKING FORM

Name: _____   School: _____

Date: _____   Skills Score %: _____

Instructions: The student receives a score of 1 for every skill demonstrated. The score is determined as a percentage of skills demonstrated divided by skills expected. Item #1 is the easiest social skill listed and item #7 is the hardest social skill.

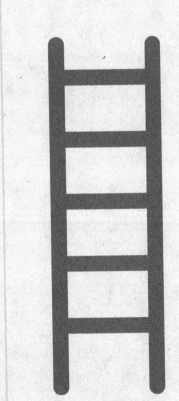

7. Demonstrates the ability to ask for help

6. Demonstrates the ability to control impulses

5. Demonstrates relevant responses to questions or comments

4. Demonstrates ability to take turns

3. Demonstrates emotions that match the situation

2. Demonstrates ability to stay on topic

1. Demonstrates empathy

Figure 4-3. Group Behaviors Data Tracking Form. (Adapted from Simmons, C. D., Griswold, L. A., & Berg, B. [2010]. Evaluation of social interaction during occupational engagement. *American Journal of Occupational Therapy, 64,* 10-17. https://doi.org/10.5014/ajot.64.1.10)

3 Taylor & Francis Group. Egan, B. E., Sears, C., & Keener, A. (Eds.). *Occupational therapy groups for addressing al health challenges in school-aged populations: A Tier 2 resource.* Taylor & Francis Group.

Motivational Behaviors Data Tracking

Student Name:_____
School:_____
Date:_____
Skills Score %:_____

Instructions: The student receives a score of 1 for every behavior demonstrated. The score is determined as a percentage of behaviors demonstrated divided by behaviors expected. Item #1 is the easiest motivational-related behavior experienced and item #10 is the most difficult motivational-related behavior experienced.

☐ 8. Seeks a Challenge

☐ 7. Invests Energy, Attention, and Emotion

☐ 6. Pursues a Task to Completion

☐ 5. Attempts to Correct Errors

☐ 4. Attempts to Solve Problems

☐ 3. Stays Engaged in Tasks

☐ 2. Initiates Tasks vs Being Told to Start

☐ 1. Shows Interest or Curiosity

Figure 4-4. Motivation Behaviors Data Tracking Form. (Adapted from Andersen, S., Kielhofner, G., & Lai, J. S. [2005]. An examination of the measurement properties of the pediatric volitional questionnaire. *Physical & Occupational Therapy in Pediatrics, 25*[1-2], 39-57.)

OCCUPATIONAL SKILLS DATA TRACKING FORM

STUDENT NAME: _____   SCHOOL:_____

DATE:_____   SKILLS SCORE %:_____

INSTRUCTIONS: THE STUDENT RECEIVES A SCORE OF 1 FOR EVERY SKILL DEMONSTRATED. THE SCORE IS DETERMINED AS A PERCENTAGE OF SKILLS DEMONSTRATED DIVIDED BY SKILLS EXPECTED. ITEM #1 IS THE EASIEST SKILL TO DEMONSTRATE AND ITEM #5 IS THE HARDEST SKILL TO DEMONSTRATE.

BASIC TASKS ___%	MANAGING LIFE & RELATIONSHIPS ___%	SATISFACTION & ACTUALIZATION ___%
☐ 5. Taking care of school responsibilities	☐ 5. Make appropriate decisions on what's important	☐ 5. Accomplish what I set out to do
☐ 4. Getting done what I need to get done	☐ 4. Involved as a member of the class	☐ 4. Working toward my goals
☐ 3. Managing basic needs	☐ 3. Identify and solve problems	☐ 3. Handling my responsibilities
☐ 2. Getting to class independently	☐ 2. Get along with others	☐ 2. Have a satisfying routine
☐ 1. Taking care of self	☐ 1. Concentrate on tasks	☐ 1. Relax and enjoy self

NOTES & OBSERVATIONS:

Figure 4-5. Occupational Skills Data Tracking Form. (Adapted from Kielhofner, G., Forsyth, K., Kramer, J., & Iyenger, A. [2009]. Developing the Occupational Self Assessment: The use of Rasch analysis to assure internal validity, sensitivity and reliability. *British Journal of Occupational Therapy, 72*[3], 94-104. https://doi.org/10.1177/030802260907200302)

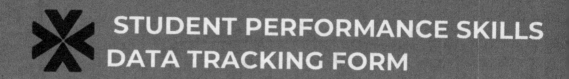

STUDENT PERFORMANCE SKILLS DATA TRACKING FORM

Student Name:_____   School:_____   Date:_____

Skills Score %:_____

Instructions: The student receives a score of 1 for every skill demonstrated. The score is determined as a percentage of skills demonstrated divided by skills expected. Item #1 is the easiest skill to demonstrate and item #6 is the hardest skill to demonstrate.

☐ 6. Attempts to solve a problem before asking for help

☐ 5. Asks for help when needed

☐ 4. Initiates work promptly

☐ 3. Recovers after failure

☐ 2. Attempts to modify performance based on constructive feedback

☐ 1. Stays on task for 15 minutes or more

Figure 4-6. Student Performance Skills Data Tracking Form. (Adapted from Hwang, J. L., & Davies, P. L. [2009]. Rasch analysis of the School Function Assessment provides additional evidence for the internal validity of the activity performance scales. *American Journal of Occupational Therapy, 63*[3], 369-373. https://doi.org/10.5014/ajot.63.3.369)

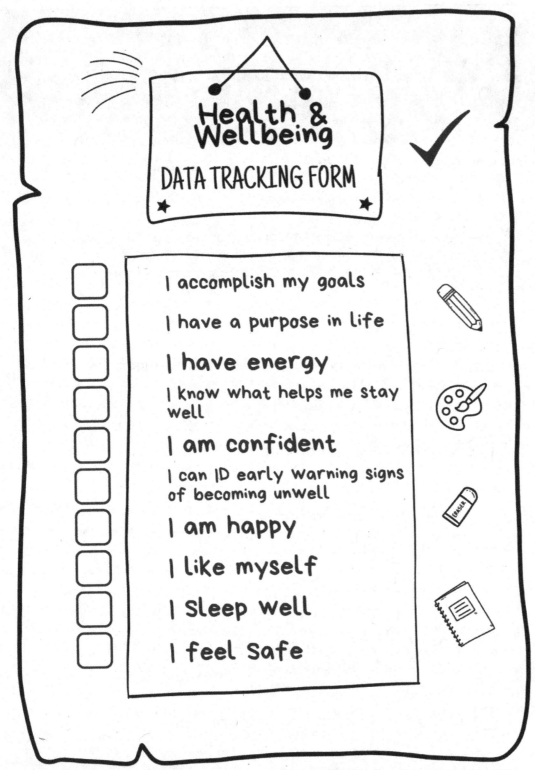

Figure 4-7. Health & Wellbeing Data Tracking Form. (Adapted from Barbic, S. P., Kidd, S. A., Durisko, Z. T., Yachouh, R., Rathitharan, G., & McKenzie, K. [2018]. What are the personal recovery needs of community-dwelling individuals with mental illness? Preliminary findings from the Canadian Personal Recovery Outcome Measurement (C-PROM) study. Canadian Journal of Community Mental Health, 37[1], 29-47. https://doi.org/10.7870/cjcmh-2018-005)

References

Andersen, S., Kielhofner, G., & Lai, J. S. (2005). An examination of the measurement properties of the pediatric vo
    questionnaire. *Physical & Occupational Therapy in Pediatrics, 25*(1-2), 39-57.

Barbic, S. P., Kidd, S. A., Durisko, Z. T., Yachouh, R., Rathitharan, G., & McKenzie, K. (2018). What are the p
    al recovery needs of community-dwelling individuals with mental illness? Preliminary findings from the Ca
    Personal Recovery Outcome Measurement (C-PROM) study. *Canadian Journal of Community Mental Health*
    29-47. https://doi.org/10.7870/cjcmh-2018-005

Hwang, J. L., & Davies, P. L. (2009). Rasch analysis of the School Function Assessment provides additional evide
    the internal validity of the activity performance scales. *American Journal of Occupational Therapy, 63*(3), 3
    https://doi.org/10.5014/ajot.63.3.369

Kielhofner, G., Forsyth, K., Kramer, J., & Iyenger, A. (2009). Developing the Occupational Self Assessment: The
    Rasch analysis to assure internal validity, sensitivity and reliability. *British Journal of Occupational Therapy, 72*
    104. https://doi.org/10.1177/030802260907200302

Simmons, C. D., Griswold, L. A., & Berg, B. (2010). Evaluation of social interaction during occupational engag
    American Journal of Occupational Therapy, 64, 10-17. https://doi.org/10.5014/ajot.64.1.10

Section 5

Additional Resources

Sample Tier 2 Letter to Parents

January 28, 2023

Dear Parent,

Hello! My name is Sally Smith, and I am the occupational therapy clinician at your child's school. In my ro[le] have the opportunity to collaborate with teachers and students at Jane Smith Elementary School to sup[port] students struggling with physical, sensory, and mental health challenges that impact their participatio[n in] expected daily school activities.

This year, I will be consulting and collaborating with administration, guidance counselors, and teacher[s in] hopes of improving student participation and success throughout the school day. Your child was rece[ntly] referred to the academic intervention team. Following a screening, they qualify for Tier 2 group support. [For] the next 8 weeks, your child will have the opportunity to participate in a weekly small group interven[tion] during nonacademic instruction. Progress will be monitored and shared. The goal of these groups is [to] provide students with the opportunity to understand positive mental health support strategies for gre[ater] success in their student role.

If you have any further questions, please reach out to your child's guidance counselor or the sch[ool] administrator.

Warm Regards,

Sally Smith, MS, OTR/L

Case Study Template

<u>Client Name</u>

STUDENT STRENGTHS   *(Identifying personal strengths is critical to promoting hope, increasing self-efficacy, and supporting recovery. To encourage continued practice with identifying strengths, the editors intentionally provided a blank three-bulleted list for each case. It is our hope that users of the resource will be able to identify even more than three strengths in each vignette.)*
OCCUPATIONAL NEEDS
SCHOOL BARRIERS: INTERNALIZING/EXTERNALIZING BEHAVIORS
PERSONAL FACTOR CONSIDERATIONS
RECOMMENDED GROUPS

Client Case Report

Group Template

GROUP TITLE	
ACTIVITY	
PURPOSE	
SESSION GOALS	
OCCUPATION AS MEANS AND ENDS	
DIRECTIONS	
MATERIALS	
MESSY FACTOR	
PINTEREST TERMS	
GRADE LEVEL	

essing the Group: Tip Sheet

troduction and Warm-Up Ideas

ays to Grade or Modify the Activity

uestions You May Want to Ask

acilitation Strategies

acilitator's Notes

If you have had success implementing these strategies and want more information to guide your practice, lowing are some helpful resources.

Education Policy

- **Every Student Succeeds Act (ESSA):** Signed by President Obama, December 10, 2015. https://www.◦ essa?src=rn
- **Individuals with Disabilities Education Act (IDEA):** Congress reauthorized the IDEA in 2004 an◦ recently amended the IDEA through Public Law 114-95, the Every Student Succeeds Act, in Decembe◦ https://sites.ed.gov/idea/about-idea/
- **National Alliance of Specialized Instructional Support Personnel (NASISP):** http://nasisp.org/
- **Rehabilitation Act of 1973; Section 504:** https://sites.ed.gov/idea/about-idea/#Rehab-Act
- **U.S. Department of Education Laws and Guidance:** https://www2.ed.gov/policy/landing.jhtml?src=◦

Relevant Articles

- Activity- and Occupation-Based Interventions to Support Mental Health, Positive Behavior, and Participation for Children and Youth: A Systematic Review
  - Cahill, S. M., Egan, B. E., & Seber, J. (2020). Activity-and occupation-based interventions to support ◦ health, positive behavior, and social participation for children and youth: A systematic review. *Am◦ Journal of Occupational Therapy, 74*(2). https://doi.org/10.5014/ajot.2020.038687
- American Occupational Therapy Association (AOTA) School Mental Health Toolkit
- AOTA Guide to Anxiety Disorders
  - American Occupational Therapy Association. (2012). Anxiety disorders. Retrieved from https://◦ aota.org/-/media/Corporate/Files/Practice/Children/SchoolMHToolkit/Anxiety%20Disorde◦ Info%20Sheet.pdf.
- AOTA Guide to Bullying Prevention and Friendship Promotion
  - American Occupational Therapy Association. (2013). Bullying prevention and friendship prom◦ Retrieved from https://www.aota.org/-/media/Corporate/Files/Practice/Children/SchoolMHT◦ BullyingPreventionInfoSheet.pdf.
- AOTA Guide to the Cafeteria: Creating a Positive Mealtime Experience
  - American Occupational Therapy Association. (2013). Creating a positive mealtime experience. Ret◦ from https://www.aota.org/-/media/Corporate/Files/Practice/Children/Cafeteria-Mealtime-Info-◦ pdf.
- AOTA Guide to Childhood Obesity
  - American Occupational Therapy Association. (2012). Childhood obesity. Retrieved from https://◦ aota.org/-/media/Corporate/Files/Practice/Children/SchoolMHToolkit/Childhood%20Obesity.pd◦
- AOTA Guide to Childhood Trauma
  - Petrenchik, T., & Weiss, D. (2015). Childhood trauma. Retrieved from https://www.aota.org/-/m◦ Corporate/Files/Practice/Children/Childhood-Trauma-Info-Sheet-2015.pdf.
- AOTA Guide to Depression
  - American Occupational Therapy Association. (2012). Depression. Retrieved from https://www◦ org/-/media/Corporate/Files/Practice/Children/SchoolMHToolkit/Depression.pdf.

OTA Guide to Foster Care

Lynch, A., Ashcraft, R., Paul-Ward, A., Tekell, L., Salamat, A., & Schefkind, S. (2017). Foster care. Retrieved from https://www.aota.org/-/media/Corporate/Files/Practice/Children/SchoolMHToolkit/Foster-Care-Info-Sheet-20170320.pdf.

OTA Guide to Grief and Loss

American Occupational Therapy Association. (2012). Grief and loss. Retrieved from https://www.aota.org/-/media/Corporate/Files/Practice/Children/SchoolMHToolkit/Grief%20and%20Loss%20Final.PDF.

OTA Guide to Inclusion of Children With Disabilities

Conway, C. S., Kanics, I. M., Mohler, R., Giudici, M. S., & Wagenfeld, A. (2015). Inclusion of children with disabilities. Retrieved from https://www.aota.org/-/media/Corporate/Files/Practice/Children/Inclusion-of-Children-With-Disabilities-20150128.PDF.

OTA Guide to Promoting Strengths in Children and Youth

American Occupational Therapy Association. (2012). Promoting strengths in children and youth. Retrieved from https://www.aota.org/-/media/Corporate/Files/Practice/Children/SchoolMHToolkit/Promoting%20Strengths%20REVISED.pdf.

OTA Guide to Recess Promotion

American Occupational Therapy Association. (2012). Recess promotion. Retrieved from https://www.aota.org/-/media/Corporate/Files/Practice/Children/SchoolMHToolkit/Recess%20Promotion.pdf.

OTA Guide to Reducing Restraint and Seclusion: The Benefit and Role of Occupational Therapy

Cahill, S. M., & Pagano, J. (2015). Reducing restraint and seclusion: The benefit and role of occupational therapy. Retrieved from https://www.aota.org/-/media/Corporate/Files/Practice/Children/Reducing-Restraint-and-Seclusion-20150218.PDF.

OTA Guide to Social and Emotional Learning

Foster, L. (2013). Social and emotional learning (SEL). Retrieved from https://www.aota.org/-/media/Corporate/Files/Practice/Children/SchoolMHToolkit/Social-and-Emotional-Learning-Info-Sheet.pdf.

OTA Occupational Therapy and School Mental Health

American Occupational Therapy Association. (2009). Occupational therapy and school mental health. AOTA Fact Sheet. https://www.aota.org/-/media/corporate/files/practice/children/browse/school/mental-health/ot%20%20school%20mental%20health%20fact%20sheet%20for%20web%20posting%20102109.pdf

OTA Tips for Educator's Successful Participation: School Strategies for All Students

Asher, A., & Lau, C. (2017). Tips for educator's successful participation: School strategies for all students. Retrieved from https://www.aota.org/-/media/Corporate/Files/AboutOT/Professionals/WhatIsOT/CY/Tips-for-Educators-Successful-Participation-School-Strategies-for-All-Students.pdf.

Expanding School-Based Problem-Solving Teams to Include Occupational Therapists

Cahill, S. M., & Lopez-Reyna, N. (2013). Expanding school-based problem-solving teams to include occupational therapists. *Journal of Occupational Therapy, Schools, & Early Intervention, 6*(4), 314-325. https://doi.org/10.1080/19411243.2013.860763

How to Use AOTA's Mental Health Information Sheets

Bazyk, S., Crabtree, L., Downing, D., Fette, C., Marr, D., Olson, L., Pizzi, M., & Schefkind, S. (2012). How to use AOTA's mental health information sheets. Retrieved from https://www.aota.org/-/media/Corporate/Files/Practice/Children/SchoolMHToolkit/How%20To%20Use%20Mental%20Health.PDF.

Identifying Youth With Mental Health Conditions at School

Cahill, S. M., & Egan, B. E. (2017). Identifying youth with mental health conditions at school. *OT Practice, 22*(5), 1-7.

- Mental Health in Children and Youth: The Benefit and Role of Occupational Therapy
  - Mahaffey, L. M. (2016). *Mental health in children and youth: The benefit and role of occupation apy*. AOTA. Retrieved from https://www.aota.org//media/Corporate/Files/AboutOT/Profess WhatIsOT/MH/Facts/MH%20in%20Children%20and%20Youth%20fact%20sheet.pdf
- Occupational Therapy's Role With School Settings
  - American Occupational Therapy Association. (2016). Occupational therapy's role with school s Retrieved from https://www.aota.org/~/media/Corporate/Files/AboutOT/Professionals/WhatIsO Fact-Sheets/School%20Settings%20fact%20sheet.pdf.

Other Resources

- 25th Annual Conference on Advancing School Mental Health, Mental Health Technology Transfer (MHTTC) Network
  - https://mhttcnetwork.org/centers/global-mhttc/25th-annual-conference-advancing-school tal-health#:~:text=The%20Annual%20Conference%20on%20Advancing%20School%20Men Health%2C,school%20mental%20health%20practice%2C%20research%2C%20training%20ai policy
- American School Counselor Association (ASCA)
  - https://www.schoolcounselor.org/
- American School Health Association
- Annual Conference, University of Maryland School of Medicine
  - https://www.schoolmentalhealth.org/Annual-Conference/
- Association for Child & Adolescent Mental Health
  - https://www.acamh.org/
- Association of Recovery Schools
  - https://recoveryschools.org/
- *Children & Schools*
- Every Moment Counts
  - https://everymomentcounts.org/
- Jackson, L., Polichino, J., & Potter, K. (2006). Transforming caseload to workload in school-based and intervention occupational therapy services. Retrieved from https://www.aota.org/-/media/Corporate AboutOT/Professionals/WhatIsOT/CY/Fact-Sheets/Workload-fact.pdf
- *Journal of Occupational Therapy, Schools, & Early Intervention*
- *Journal of School Health*
  - https://onlinelibrary.wiley.com/journal/17461561
- Motivational Interviewing
  - https://motivationalinterviewing.org/understanding-motivational-interviewing
- National Alliance on Mental Illness, Mental Health in Schools
  - https://www.nami.org/Advocacy/Policy-Priorities/Improving-Health/Mental-Health-in-Schools
- National Association of School Psychologist (NASP)
  - https://www.nasponline.org/
- National Center for School Mental Health Resources–SHAPE System
  - https://www.schoolmentalhealth.org/Resources/
- National Center on Safe Supportive Learning Environments (NCSSLE)
  - https://safesupportivelearning.ed.gov/topic-research/school-climate-measurement/school-clii survey-compendium

National Child Traumatic Stress Network (NCTSN)
  https://www.nctsn.org/
School Mental Health: A Multidisciplinary Research and Practice Journal
School Social Work Association of America (SSWAA)
  https://www.sswaa.org/
School Social Work Network (SSWN)
  https://schoolsocialwork.net/
Society of Clinical Child and Adolescent Psychology
  https://sccap53.org/
UCLA School Mental Health Project
  http://smhp.psych.ucla.edu/
U.S. Department of Education, Office of Safe and Supportive Schools
  https://oese.ed.gov/offices/office-of-formula-grants/safe-supportive-schools/
Youth.Gov, School-Based Mental Health
  https://youth.gov/youth-topics/youth-mental-health/school-based

Financial Disclosures

Dr. Molly Bathje has no financial or proprietary interest in the materials presented herein.

Dr. Patricia Bowyer has no financial or proprietary interest in the materials presented herein.

Stephanie Brauch has no financial or proprietary interest in the materials presented herein.

Anna Brown has no financial or proprietary interest in the materials presented herein.

Mark Bumgarner has no financial or proprietary interest in the materials presented herein.

Dr. Susan Cahill has no financial or proprietary interest in the materials presented herein.

Dr. Bobbi Carrlson has no financial or proprietary interest in the materials presented herein.

Dr. Theresa Carlson Carroll has no financial or proprietary interest in the materials presented herein.

Ray Cendejas has no financial or proprietary interest in the materials presented herein.

Dr. Paula Cook has no financial or proprietary interest in the materials presented herein.

Marcela De La Pava has no financial or proprietary interest in the materials presented herein.

Dr. Anna Domina has no financial or proprietary interest in the materials presented herein.

Jerry Dye, Jr. has no financial or proprietary interest in the materials presented herein.

Dr. Megan Eads has no financial or proprietary interest in the materials presented herein.

Dr. Brad E. Egan has no financial or proprietary interest in the materials presented herein.

Dr. Caitlin Esposito has no financial or proprietary interest in the materials presented herein.

Dr. Ashley Fecht has no financial or proprietary interest in the materials presented herein.

Dr. Susan Friuglietti has no financial or proprietary interest in the materials presented herein.

Renee Harris has no financial or proprietary interest in the materials presented herein.

Dr. Jenna L. Heffron has no financial or proprietary interest in the materials presented herein.

Kelsey Helgesen has no financial or proprietary interest in the materials presented herein.

Financial Disclosures

Iettlinger has no financial or proprietary interest in the materials presented herein.

y Wilson James has no financial or proprietary interest in the materials presented herein.

t S. Jedlicka has no financial or proprietary interest in the materials presented herein.

n Keener has no financial or proprietary interest in the materials presented herein.

e Kiraly-Alvarez has no financial or proprietary interest in the materials presented herein.

istine Kivlen has no financial or proprietary interest in the materials presented herein.

a LeFlore has no financial or proprietary interest in the materials presented herein.

hryn M. Loukas has no financial or proprietary interest in the materials presented herein.

nda Mahoney has no financial or proprietary interest in the materials presented herein.

y (Tony) Mesiano, Jr. has no financial or proprietary interest in the materials presented herein.

ah Nielsen has no financial or proprietary interest in the materials presented herein.

e Clifford O'Brien has no financial or proprietary interest in the materials presented herein.

Ochoa has an endorsement agreement with Rhythm Band Instruments where he receives free and/or
nted items.

urette Olson has no financial or proprietary interest in the materials presented herein.

nda M. Olson has no financial or proprietary interest in the materials presented herein.

na Rainelli has no financial or proprietary interest in the materials presented herein.

ashauna (Neki) Richardson has no financial or proprietary interest in the materials presented herein.

. Rupp has no financial or proprietary interest in the materials presented herein.

in Schwier has no financial or proprietary interest in the materials presented herein.

ndy Sears has no financial or proprietary interest in the materials presented herein.

ubrey Sejuit has no financial or proprietary interest in the materials presented herein.

han Smeraglia has no financial or proprietary interest in the materials presented herein.

Dr. Pam Stephenson has no financial or proprietary interest in the materials presented herein.

Dr. Ashley Stoffel has no financial or proprietary interest in the materials presented herein.

Dr. Karen Stornello has no financial or proprietary interest in the materials presented herein.

Dr. Meghan Suman has no financial or proprietary interest in the materials presented herein.

Dr. Andrea Thinnes has no financial or proprietary interest in the materials presented herein.

Dr. Ryan Thomure has no financial or proprietary interest in the materials presented herein.

Dr. Patricia (Patee) Tomsic has no financial or proprietary interest in the materials presented herein.

Dr. Ingris Treminio has no financial or proprietary interest in the materials presented herein.

Jeaneen M. Tucker has no financial or proprietary interest in the materials presented herein.

Dr. Jessica Weiler has no financial or proprietary interest in the materials presented herein.

Index

Index

n the United States
& Taylor Publisher Services